H
M
th

How to Master the BMAT

Unbeatable preparation for success in the BioMedical Admissions Test

Dr Christopher See
Dr Chris Tyreman

3rd edition

KoganPage

LONDON PHILADELPHIA NEW DELHI

First published in Great Britain and the United States in 2009 by Kogan Page Limited
Second edition 2011
Reprinted 2012 (three times)
Third edition 2015

2nd Floor, 45 Gee Street	1518 Walnut Street, Suite 1100	4737/23 Ansari Road
London EC1V 3RS	Philadelphia PA 19102	Daryaganj
United Kingdom	USA	New Delhi 110002
www.koganpage.com		India

© Dr Chris Tyreman, 2009, 2011
© Dr Christopher See and Dr Chris Tyreman, 2015

The right of Dr Christopher See and Dr Chris Tyreman to be identified as the author of this work has been asserted by them in accordance with the Copyright, Designs and Patents Act 1988.

ISBN   978 0 7494 7187 3
E-ISBN 978 0 7494 7188 0

British Library Cataloguing-in-Publication Data

A CIP record for this book is available from the British Library.

Library of Congress Cataloging-in-Publication Data

Tyreman, C. J., author.
   How to master the BMAT : unbeatable preparation for success in the biomedical admissions test / Chris Tyreman, Christopher See. – Third edition.
      p. ; cm.
   ISBN 978-0-7494-7187-3 – ISBN 978-0-7494-7188-0 (e-ISBN)
   I. See, Christopher, author. II. Title.
   [DNLM: 1. Education, Medical–Great Britain–Examination Questions.   W 18.2]
   R772
   610.71'141–dc23
                                                            2014046781

Typeset by Graphicraft Limited, Hong Kong
Print production managed by Jellyfish
Printed and bound by CPI Group (UK) Ltd, Croydon CR0 4YY

Contents

Introduction 1

PART ONE
Reviews 5

1   Aptitude and skills review 7

A1. Understanding argument 1: basic aspects 7
A2. Understanding argument 2: flaws; types of questions 8
A3. Understanding argument 3: example argument 10
A4. Critical thinking: Venn diagrams and logic statements 11
A5. Shape symmetry 12
Aptitude review questions 13

2   Maths review 16

M1.   Mental arithmetic review 1: basic operations 17
M2.   Mental arithmetic review 2: further operations 18
M3.   Fractions 1: basic arithmetic 19
M4.   Fractions 2: improper fractions; ratios 20
M5.   Decimals 1: fraction/decimal conversions and basic arithmetic 21
M6.   Decimals 2: rounding (decimal place, significant figure) and standard form 22
M7.   Per cent (%) 23
M8.   Time and clocks 25
M9.   Areas, perimeters, volumes and surface area 26
M10.   Algebra 1: substitution and re-arranging 27
M11.   Algebra 2: simultaneous and quadratic equations 29
M12.   Averages: mean, median, mode; weighted 30
M13.   Pie and bar charts, line and scatter graphs, tables 31
M14.   Cumulative frequency, box and whisker plots 32
M15.   Geometry 1: angles and lines, triangles, other shapes 34
M16.   Geometry 2: Pythagoras and trigonometric functions 35

M17. Circle theorems 36

M18. Inequalities 37

M19. Probability 1: basic concepts 38

M20. Probability 2: tree diagrams 39

M21. Permutations and combinations 40

Maths review questions 42

3   Physics review 48

P1. Measurements and prefixes 49

P2. Conventions for units, symbols and numbers 50

P3. SI base units for length, volume, mass 50

P4. Equations of motion 51

P5. Graphs of motion 52

P6. Projectile motion 53

P7. Force and motion (Newton) 54

P8. Force, work, power and energy 55

P9. Universal gravitation, satellites and escape velocity 55

P10. Force, momentum and impulse 56

P11. Force, stress and strain 57

P12. Moments, mechanical advantage, levers and pulleys 58

P13. Pressure, buoyancy and flow 59

P14. Gas laws 59

P15. Heat and energy 60

P16. Waves (light and sound) 61

P17. Electrostatics, capacitance and electricity 62

P18. Kirchhoff's circuit laws, resistors and capacitors 63

P19. Electromagnetism and electromagnetic induction 64

P20. Radioactive decay 65

Physics review questions 66

4   Chemistry review 70

C1. Atoms, electron configuration and valency 70

C2. Periodic table 72

C3. Bonding: electrovalent (ionic), covalent and metallic 72

C4. The mole and balancing chemical equations (reactions) 73

C5. Types of chemical reaction 74

C6. Concentration and pH; reaction rates 76

C7. Exothermic and endothermic reactions; Le Chatelier's principle 77

C8. Solids, liquids, gases; changes of state; thermochemistry 78

C9. Electrochemistry, reactivity series and electrolysis 79

C10. Carbon (organic) chemistry; fractional distillation 80
Chemistry review questions 82

5 Biology review 87

B1. Digestive system 87
B2. Respiratory system 88
B3. Circulatory system 89
B4. Nervous system; eye 90
B5. Endocrine system; menstrual cycle hormones 91
B6. Urinary system 92
B7. DNA (deoxyribonucleic acid), genes and cell division 94
B8. Patterns of inheritance 95
Biology review questions 98

6 Writing task review 102

W1. Choice of question 102
W2. Preparation 103
W3. The four-paragraph approach 103
W4. Composing the essay 104
W5. Sources and resources 105
W6. The final check 107
Instructions for mock tests 111

PART TWO
Tests and answers 113

7 Mock tests 115

Mock Test 1: Aptitude and skills 115
Mock Test 2: Scientific knowledge and applications 131
Mock Test 3: Writing task 141
Mock Test 4: Aptitude and skills 142
Mock Test 5: Scientific knowledge and applications 159
Mock Test 6: Writing task 171
Mock Test 7: Aptitude and skills 172
Mock Test 8: Scientific knowledge and applications 188
Mock Test 9: Writing task 199
Mock Test 10: Aptitude and skills 200
Mock Test 11: Scientific knowledge and applications 218
Mock Test 12: Writing task 230

Mock Test 13: Aptitude and skills 231
Mock Test 14: Scientific knowledge and applications 251
Mock Test 15: Writing task 262

8   Answers and explanations 263

Answers to review questions 263
Answers to mock tests 268

Introduction

Use this book to boost your BMAT score

This book will maximize your BioMedical Admissions Test (BMAT) score in the shortest time with the least possible effort. It focuses on the core knowledge in the six key skill areas. There are no chapters dealing with interviews or why you want to be a doctor/vet. Written in a note-taking style, it is easy to pick up and revise without being off-putting due to passages of time-consuming text or wordiness.

Fifty per cent revision, fifty per cent practice

The book is complete in two halves. The first half, of about 100 pages, consists of six sections of revision material for the Maths, Physics, Chemistry and Biology components of the BMAT, with additional notes for problem solving and the writing task. At the end of each section, a set of review questions enables you to identify and improve your weak areas before you sit the test. The second half, also of about 100 pages, consists of practice papers that reflect the BMAT test. Candidates are supported throughout the book, and where possible every question comes complete with its revision topics indicated in brackets; for example (P3b; M6d) means revise Physics topic 3b and Maths topics 6d to answer the question; (B1a; C10b,c) means revise Biology topic 1a and Chemistry topics 10b and 10c.

No other book is required

Do not worry if, for example, you dropped Physics or Chemistry two years ago. With this 'all-in-one book' you can fill in the gaps in your knowledge without having to buy any other books. Even if a subject is new to you, rapid progress is possible because the level of prior knowledge is assumed to be low.

Expanded answers

Some other books provide only a 'right/wrong' marking scheme, which is fine if you have chosen the correct answer but is otherwise of limited help. In this book, almost every question comes with an expanded answer that offers sufficient explanation as to the method involved.

Hints to the solution

It is often the case that a *clue* to the method of answer serves to jog the memory. For this reason, many of the questions include a *hint* as to the solution. Even so, candidates should try to answer the question without referring to the hint (written below the answer choices) in the first instance. For some candidates the hint will 'give the game away', though in many instances it will not and in any case the solution may still be several steps away. This method of learning is an aid to memory and reduces the chances of 'getting stuck' and then having to turn to the answer as the only means forward.

BMAT test format

The Biomedical Admissions Test lasts two hours. It has three sections and the first two are marked by computer. No calculators or dictionaries are permitted.

Section 1: Aptitude and skills: 35 multiple-choice or short-answer questions; time allowed one hour.

Section 2: Scientific knowledge and applications: 27 multiple-choice or short-answer questions; time allowed 30 minutes.

Section 3: Writing task: answer one question from a choice of three; one side of A4 paper; time allowed 30 minutes.

BMAT registration

Entry to the BioMedical Admissions Test is via Cambridge Assessment. Full details of how and where to sit the BMAT are available on the BMAT website: http://www.bmat.org.uk. The test is taken in November and the deadline for standard applications is at the end of September.

A list of universities/courses requiring the BMAT can be found on the UCAS website: http://www.ucas.ac.uk. At the time of writing, the BMAT is taken by students wishing to read medicine, veterinary medicine and related courses at the University of Oxford, the University of Cambridge, Imperial College London, University College London and the Royal Veterinary College.

Reviews

CHAPTER 1

Aptitude and skills review

A1.   Understanding argument 1: basic aspects
A2.   Understanding argument 2: flaws; types of questions
A3.   Understanding argument 3: example argument
A4.   Critical thinking: Venn diagrams and logic statements
A5.   Shape symmetry
        Aptitude review questions

A1. Understanding argument 1: basic aspects

a) Argument

An argument is a short passage of prose that usually contains a *conclusion* and the *evidence* (reasons) supporting it. The evidence is presented in one or more *premises* (statements) that appear plausible within the context of the argument. A conclusion is often expressed at the end of the passage or at the beginning, and its *validity* depends upon: i) the truth of the premises, including any *assumptions* that the reader is expected to take for granted, and ii) the soundness of the reasoning from the evidence to the conclusion.

b) Conclusion, evidence and assumptions

i)   **The conclusion** is a judgement based on reasoning from premises; the following words are indicators: therefore, consequently, in summary, so, hence, infer, shows, should, will.

ii) **The evidence** is the knowledge required to support the conclusion; the following words are indicators: obviously, because, for example, in support of, due to, since, as a result of.

iii) **The assumptions** provide the link between the evidence and the conclusion as long as they are true. Assumptions are not stated but are deemed to 'go without saying'; in other words, proof is not given, so you have to read between the lines.

c) Reasoning

i)   **Deductive:** the conclusion is deduced from generally accepted facts and a minor premise. For example: all planets orbit the sun; Mars is a planet so Mars must orbit the sun.

ii) **Inductive** (most arguments): the conclusion is drawn from minor premises (ie *inferred* from observation and patterns) that are believed to support the general case of something (eg a theory) but do not provide *conclusive* proof; for example, Mars moves around the sun and the earth moves around the sun so the sun is at the centre of all the planets (*probable*). There are three key possibilities: the conclusion is true with true premises and sound (valid) reasoning; the conclusion is false with sound reasoning (but false premises); the conclusion is false with true premises (but unsound reasoning).

A2. Understanding argument 2: flaws; types of questions

a) Flaws

These are errors in arguments leading to misleading or unsafe conclusions:

● Confusing correlation with causation. For example, death rates are higher in cancer patients receiving complementary therapies, so complementary therapies must be harmful to health (untrue: when orthodox medicine fails, patients are more seriously ill).

- Confusion over percentages and numbers. For example, 15 per cent of road fatalities involve motorbikes and 75 per cent involve cars so it is five times safer to ride a motorbike than to drive a car (untrue: fewer than one in 50 vehicles are motorbikes).

- Over-generalizing. For example, nine out of 10 people interviewed said they would buy a small car next time so there is little market for the large car (sample too small or unrepresentative; all those interviewed drove small cars).

- Logical fallacy: the premises are true but do not support the conclusion (though it may be true). For example, if A follows B (true) then so must C, D and E (false). Note that a true conclusion can be arrived at (accidentally) with false premises.

b) Question types

Questions in the BMAT take various forms:

- A short paragraph that contains a conclusion and the evidence that supports it. You should assume that the evidence (premises) is true for the purposes of the argument; ie, do not introduce your own knowledge base or opinions. Choose an answer that:
  - is the *best conclusion* (ie the main thrust of the argument or what can be safely *inferred*), or
  - identifies what has been *implied* (not directly stated or assumed, but suggested or hinted at), or
  - identifies what *must be assumed* for the conclusion to hold true, or
  - would *weaken* the argument if it were true (ie contradictory statement; alternative explanation), or
  - would *strengthen* the argument if it were true (ie supportive statement; consistent), or
  - would show the conclusion to be untrue (eg a *fallacy*).

Read every answer choice before selecting the best response.

- A longer passage of more than one paragraph followed by three questions designed to check reading comprehension; numerical data may be included.

A3. Understanding argument 3: example argument

Argument: Motorway speed limits should be increased to 80 mph. The current limit of 70 mph was introduced in 1965 when cars were less well engineered than today. Modern cars are designed for speeds well in excess of 80 mph so there is no need to restrict motorway speeds to 70 mph.

Conclusion: Motorway speed limits should be increased to 80 mph.
Evidence (taken as fact): Modern cars are better engineered.
Evidence (taken as fact): They are designed for speeds well over 80 mph.
Assumption (can be challenged): Driving at 80 mph is safe if the car is designed to do it.

The above argument can be weakened by contradictory evidence or strengthened by supportive evidence. For example:

- *Significantly weakening*: It may be the case that motor vehicle accidents on motorways usually involve speeds in excess of the current limit (challenges a questionable assumption).

- *Significantly strengthening*: It may be the case that most accidents are not caused by speeding (supports 70 mph+).

- *Slightly weakening*: It may be the case that higher speeds lead to more serious accidents (true but outside scope of argument).

- *Slightly strengthening*: It may be the case that there have been major improvements in highway engineering since 1965 (true but outside scope of argument).

- *Inference*: Increasing the motorway speed limit to 80 mph will not lead to more accidents (main thrust of argument).

- *Irrelevant*: Carbon dioxide emissions will increase if the speed limit is raised (true but outside scope of argument).

A4. Critical thinking: Venn diagrams and logic statements

a) Venn diagrams

For example: 48 patients attend a chest clinic; 29 have asthma (A), 30 have bronchitis (B) and 8 have neither disease. How many patients have both asthma and bronchitis? Method: draw a rectangle (*universal set*) containing two overlapping circles A and B.

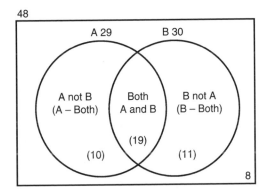

(A not B) + Both = 29; (B not A) + Both = 30; add to give:

1) (A not B) + (B not A) + 2 × Both = 59
2) (A not B) + (B not A) + Both = 48 − 8 = 40

1) − 2) gives Both = 19

Summary: A only = 10; B only = 11;
both A and B = 19; A + B + Both = 40; neither = 8.

b) Logic statements

Logic statements are two premises that lead to a conclusion. For example:

1. All cattle are animals.
2. All bulls are cattle.
3. Therefore all bulls are animals.

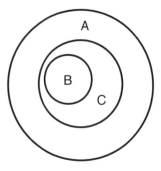

(NB: this is a logic statement diagram, not a Venn diagram)

A5. Shape symmetry

a) Reflection symmetry

Reflection symmetry is also known as line symmetry; it occurs where a shape appears identical, or symmetrical, either side of a line, as in a mirror image. Shapes can have one, two or more lines of symmetry, for example:

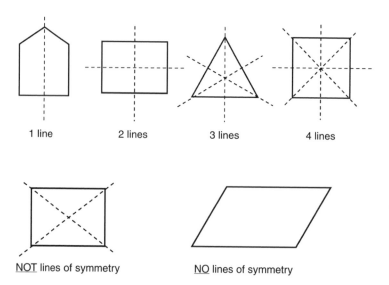

1 line   2 lines   3 lines   4 lines

NOT lines of symmetry   NO lines of symmetry

b) Rotational symmetry

A shape has rotational symmetry if it can be rotated about its centre and still look the same. A square has four orders of rotational symmetry (90°, 180°, 270°, 360°).

| 0 orders | 2 orders | 3 orders | 4 orders |

Aptitude review questions

Q1 (A2, 3) The nuclear industry claims that its power stations are safe and no threat to people. If this is true, then why do they locate their power plants away from population centres? By doing so they are admitting that nuclear power is potentially dangerous to local communities.

Which one of the following, if true, would most seriously weaken the above argument?

A. Reactors are located away from communities as part of a general risk management strategy.
B. The potential for harm following any leak is significantly reduced.
C. Cooling water for the reactors is not available in populated areas.
D. Costs are lower and local communities are less likely to oppose planning applications.

Answer ▢

Q2 (A2, 3) Bio-diesel is not an alternative to petroleum-based diesel in the fight against carbon dioxide emissions from car exhausts; carbon is carbon and when it burns it produces carbon dioxide. The source of the carbon does not influence the size of the carbon footprint.

Which one of the following, if true, would significantly weaken the above argument?

A. Bio-fuel crops fix carbon dioxide during photosynthesis.
B. Bio-diesel accounts for less than 5 per cent of diesel combusted.
C. Cars are not the major source of carbon dioxide emissions.
D. Carbon-dioxide-fixing rainforest is cut down to make way for bio-diesel crops.

Answer ▢

Q3   (A2, 3) Clinically obese patients, ie those with a Body Mass Index (BMI) of more than 30, should be denied knee-joint surgery. The risk of complications following surgery is too great and the new joint is more likely to fail under the load.

Which two of the following, if true, would most weaken the above argument?

A. Joint life is only reduced in the morbidly obese (BMI > 40).
B. Clinically obese patients are entitled to treatment just as much as anyone else.
C. Obesity is a significant risk factor for osteoarthritis.
D. General health is more important than clinical obesity where complications are concerned.
E. It would be better if clinically obese patients were made to lose weight before they underwent joint surgery.

Answer

Q4   (A2, 3) ACE-inhibitors, beta-blockers, calcium-channel blockers and diuretics are the four main classes of drugs used to lower high blood pressure. However, in a randomized controlled trial (RCT) drinking beetroot juice was found to be equally effective in reducing blood pressure. These findings offer an alternative method of controlling hypertension.

Which two of the following, if true, would seriously weaken the above argument?

A. The participants consumed a large volume of beetroot juice.
B. Beetroot juice is an effective diuretic.
C. The control group drank water.
D. None of the participants had high blood pressure.
E. Reducing dietary salt and eating more green leafy vegetables also helps to reduce high blood pressure.

Answer

Q5   (A2, 3) Building offshore wind turbines on a massive scale is not the best way to cut carbon emissions. The money saved by not building them could be directed towards energy efficiency savings in the home. Some council properties have been supplied with free, energy-saving incandescent light-bulbs. These use 80 per cent less electricity, producing 25 kg less carbon dioxide per year. Supplying every household with three incandescent bulbs will save more energy than the UK's target for energy to be supplied by wind power.

Statement: Traditional light-bulbs are an obsolete technology and should be phased out, but the UK needs a diverse range of modern technologies to combat climate change.

Which of the following best describes how the short statement relates to the argument?

A. It refutes the argument entirely.
B. It lends qualified support for the argument.
C. It summarizes the main point of the argument.
D. It neither supports nor refutes the argument.
E. It is largely irrelevant to the main points of the argument.

Answer _____

Q6   Place the following four sentences in the order in which they form the most coherent passage.

A. Originally, being politically correct meant avoiding ideas or language that might offend minority groups.
B. Not infrequently this viewpoint is enforced by a politically correct majority that has not even consulted the minority it purports to support.
C. Political correctness has steadily chipped away at our freedom of speech.
D. More recently it has been seen as tolerating only one viewpoint that is deemed to be acceptable or true.

Answer _____

CHAPTER 2

Maths review

M1.	Mental arithmetic review 1: basic operations
M2.	Mental arithmetic review 2: further operations
M3.	Fractions 1: basic arithmetic
M4.	Fractions 2: improper fractions; ratios
M5.	Decimals 1: fraction/decimal conversions and basic arithmetic
M6.	Decimals 2: rounding (decimal place, significant figure) and standard form
M7.	Per cent (%)
M8.	Time and clocks
M9.	Areas, perimeters, volumes and surface area
M10.	Algebra 1: substitution and re-arranging
M11.	Algebra 2: simultaneous and quadratic equations
M12.	Averages: mean, median, mode; weighted
M13.	Pie and bar charts, line and scatter graphs, tables
M14.	Cumulative frequency, box and whisker plots
M15.	Geometry 1: angles and lines, triangles, other shapes
M16.	Geometry 2: Pythagoras and trigonometric functions
M17.	Circle theorems
M18.	Inequalities
M19.	Probability 1: basic concepts

M20.   Probability 2: tree diagrams
M21.   Permutations and combinations
        Maths review questions

M1. Mental arithmetic review 1: basic operations

Calculators are not allowed in the BMAT, so memorize the mental arithmetic table.

	1	2	3	4	5	6	7	8	9
1	1	2	3	4	5	6	7	8	9
2	2	4	6	8	10	12	14	16	18
3	3	6	9	12	15	18	21	24	27
4	4	8	12	16	20	24	28	32	36
5	5	10	15	20	25	30	35	40	45
6	6	12	18	24	30	36	42	48	54
7	7	14	21	28	35	42	49	56	63
8	8	16	24	32	40	48	56	64	72
9	9	18	27	36	45	54	63	72	81

For the purposes of the BMAT, mental arithmetic means with a pen and paper, so write down as many steps as you need to in a calculation to minimize the chance of making a careless mistake. All you want is the correct answers; impressive mental arithmetic counts for very little. Use 'place values':

Example: $7532 + 4316 = 7 + 4(\times 1000) + 5 + 3(\times 100) + 3 + 1(\times 10) + 8$

Write down $= 11\,000 + 800 + 48$

Similarly: $7532 \times 3 = 21\,000 + 1500 + 90 + 6 = 22\,500 + 96 = 22\,596$

Division: $456 \div 12 = (480 \div 12) - (24 \div 12) = 40 - 2 = 38$

The following rules are helpful when dividing:

i)   If the last digit is 0, 2, 4, 6 or 8, the number will divide by 2.
ii)   If the last digit ends in 0 or 5, the number will divide by 5.
iii) If the last digit ends in 0, the number will divide by 10.
iv)   If the last two digits divide by 4, the number will divide by 4.

Factorize large numbers (useful for cancelling fractions) by dividing them by prime numbers (2, 3, 5, 7, 11, 13 etc). Example: $504 = 2 \times 2 \times 2 \times 3 \times 3 \times 7$.

M2. Mental arithmetic review 2: further operations

a) Negative numbers

Addition: $(-2) + 6 = 4$; $2 + (-6) = -4$; $(-2) + (-6) = -8$.
Subtraction: $(-2) - 6 = -8$; $2 - (-6) = 8$; $(-2) - (-6) = 4$.
Multiplication: $2 \times (-6) = -12$; $(-2) \times 6 = -12$; $(-2) \times (-6) = 12$.
Division $6 \div (-3) = -2$; $(-6) \div 3 = -2$; $(-6) \div (-3) = 2$.

b) BIDMAS = Order of working out problems (first to last)

B = Brackets.
I = Indices.
D = Division.
M = Multiplication.
A = Addition.
S = Subtraction.

Example: $(35 + 15) \times 2^2 + 10 \times 14 - 480 \div 3$

Work from left to right obeying the BIDMAS rules:

$50 \times 4 + 140 - 160 = 200 - 20 = 180$

c) Index laws

i) **examples of using indices (with powers of 10):**
$10^5 \times 10^2 = 10^7$; $10^5 \div 10^2 = 10^3$; $(10^3)^2 = 10^6$; $10^{-6} = 1/10^6$;
$10^{1/2} \times 10^{1/2} = 10^1 = 10$ (ie $10^{1/2} = \sqrt{10}$); $10^0 = 1$.

ii) **surds:** eg $\sqrt{12} = \sqrt{4} \times \sqrt{3} = 2\sqrt{3}$; $\sqrt{10} \div \sqrt{5} = \sqrt{10/5} = \sqrt{2}$.

iii) **logarithm:** if $x = b^y$ then $\log_b x = y$ by definition; examples are: $100 = 10^2$ then $\log_{10} 100 = 2$ (log to the base 10 of 100 = 2); $32 = 2^5$ then $\log_2 32 = 5$ (log to the base 2 of 32 = 5); also note that $\log_b x + \log_b y = \log_b (xy)$ so $\log_b 100 + \log_b 100\ 000$;

$= 2 + 6 = \log_b(10^8)$; in other words, add log values when multiplying numbers and subtract log values when dividing numbers.

d) Factors

Factors divide into other numbers exactly without leaving a remainder. For instance, the factors of 24 are: 1 and 24, 2 and 12, 3 and 8, 4 and 6 (ie 1, 2, 3, 4, 6, 8, 12 and 24); the factors of 15 are: 1 and 15, 3 and 5 (ie 1, 3, 5 and 15). The highest *common factor* (HCF) of 24 and 15 is 3. Factors are used for breaking down large numbers and for cancelling fractions.

e) Progressions (trends)

i) **Arithmetic series:** consecutive numbers increase or decrease in value by the *common difference* (d), eg 6, 9, 12, 15, 18, $d = 3$; for an initial value of a the formula is: $a + (a + d) + (a + 2d) \ldots n^{\text{th}}$ term $= (a + (n - 1)d)$; eg 25th term is $6 + 24 \times 3 = 78$; sum of series $S_n = n \times$ (first + last)/2

ii) **Geometric series:** consecutive numbers increase or decrease in value by a constant factor known as the *common ratio* (r) eg 4, 20, 100, 500, 2500; common ratio $r = 5$; the formula is $a + ar^2 + ar^3 + ar^4 + ar^5$ and the nth term is ar^{n-1}; for instance, in the above series the 8th term is 4×5^7; sum of series $S^n = a1(1-r^n) / (1-r^n)$ where $S =$ sum to the nth terms [or n'th partial sum], a1 is the first term and r is the common ratio.

iii) **letters** may be used in place of numbers; for example $A = 1$, $B = 2$, $C = 3$, $D = 4$ etc.

M3. Fractions 1: basic arithmetic

a) Fractions

Fractions: cancel (simplify) fractions by dividing the numerator and the denominator by the same *prime factors* (2, 3, 5, 7, 11, 13 etc), starting with the smallest (2) to give the *equivalent fractions*. Example:

$$\text{eg } \frac{72}{180} = \frac{36}{90} = \frac{18}{45} = \frac{6}{15} = \frac{2}{5} \text{ (divide by 2, 2, 3, and 3)}$$

i) **Addition/subtraction of fractions:** if the denominators are the same, write the denominator once and add/subtract the two top numbers.

eg $\dfrac{5}{7} + \dfrac{3}{7} = \dfrac{8}{7} = 1\dfrac{1}{7}$ If the denominators are different, find a common denominator that both denominators will divide into.

eg $\dfrac{5}{6} + \dfrac{3}{8}$ The most obvious common denominator is 48 (6×8). However, the lowest common denominator (LCD) is 24. It makes the working out easier and can be found by comparing equivalent fractions.

ii) **Multiplication/division of fractions:** for multiplication, multiply the two numerators together and the two denominators together.

eg $\dfrac{5}{6} \times \dfrac{7}{10} = \dfrac{5 \times 7}{6 \times 10} = \dfrac{35}{60} = \dfrac{7}{12}$; alternatively you can cross-cancel the 5 and 10 as

a first step: $\dfrac{1}{6} \times \dfrac{7}{2}$ and then multiply.

iii) **Division:** similar to multiplication except that the fraction on the right-hand side is turned upside down and then multiplied by the fraction on the left-hand side.

eg $\dfrac{5}{6} \div \dfrac{7}{10}$ becomes $\dfrac{5}{6} \times \dfrac{10}{7}$; cancelling 6 and 10 by 2 gives

$\dfrac{5}{3} \times \dfrac{5}{7} = \dfrac{25}{21} = 1\dfrac{4}{21}$ (1 whole $= \dfrac{21}{21}$)

M4. Fractions 2: improper fractions; ratios

a) Improper fractions

Improper fractions (numerator greater than the denominator) are added, subtracted, multiplied and divided in exactly the same way as for proper fractions. The answer shown below is a *mixed number* containing both a whole number and a fraction.

eg $\dfrac{7}{4} - \dfrac{1}{8} = \dfrac{14}{8} - \dfrac{1}{8} = \dfrac{13}{8} = 1\dfrac{5}{8}$

Mixed numbers are added and subtracted by keeping the whole numbers and the fractions separate, and multiplied and divided by converting to improper fractions.

eg $1\dfrac{1}{8} \times 2\dfrac{3}{4} + 1\dfrac{7}{8} = \dfrac{9}{8} \times \dfrac{11}{4} + 1\dfrac{7}{8} = \dfrac{99}{32} + 1\dfrac{7}{8} = 3\dfrac{3}{32} + 1\dfrac{7}{8} = 3\dfrac{3}{32} + 1\dfrac{28}{32} = 4\dfrac{31}{32}$

b) Ratios

Ratios are similar to fractions with the whole divided into parts. Example: divide 80 in the ratio 3:1.

1st step: work out the number of parts in the whole, in this case: 3 + 1 = 4 (four quarters).
2nd step: work out the proportional parts (the fractions); these are 3/4 and 1/4.
3rd step: multiply the whole by the proportional parts: 3/4 × 80 = 60; 1/4 × 80 = 20 (check: 60 + 20 = 80).

Ratios can be simplified in the same way as fractions by cancelling both sides by a common factor (by 2, 3 etc).
Example: The ratio of boys to girls in a class of 36 is 20:16. Express this ratio in its simplest terms.
20:16 = 10:8 = 5:4 (five boys for every four girls).

M5. Decimals 1: fraction/decimal conversions and basic arithmetic

a) Fractions to decimals and vice versa

i) **Fraction to decimal:** re-write as a division; eg 3/25 re-write as 25 into 3.00.

$$ie \quad 25 \overline{)3.00} \quad \overset{12}{}$$

ii) **Decimal to fraction:** use place values; eg 0.6 = 6 tenths = 6/10 = 3/5;
0.004 = 4 thousandths = 4/1000 = 1/250.

Equivalent fractions of the more common decimals:
eg 0.25 = one-quarter; 0.5 = one-half; 0.75 = three-quarters.
0.1 = one-tenth; 0.2 = one-fifth; 0.125 = one-eighth; 0.375 = three-eighths.
0.01 = one-hundredth; 0.005 = five-thousandths.

b) Basic arithmetic

i) **Addition and subtraction:** maintain place values:
eg 0.5 + 0.043 + 0.00021 = 0.54321.

ii) **Multiplication:** for multiples (powers) of 10 the decimal point is moved to the right by the respective number of zeros.

eg $0.95 \times 10 = 9.5$ $0.95 \times 100 = 95$ $0.95 \times 1000 = 950$.

For numbers other than 10 you ignore the decimal point and then add it back in using the following rule:

Decimal places in the question = decimal places in the answer.

For example 8×10.75, ignore the decimal point:

$8 \times 1075 = 8 \times 1000 + 8 \times 75 = 8000 + 4 \times 150 = 8600$.

Number of decimal places = 2; ie 8600 becomes 86.00.

(NB check magnitude: 8×10.75 is approximately $8 \times 11 = 88$.)

iii) **division:** reverse of multiplication for multiples (powers) of 10: move the decimal point to the left.

$40.75 \div 10 = 4.075$; $\div 100 = 0.4075$; $\div 1000 = 0.04075$.

Division of or by decimal numbers can be facilitated by using a multiplication step to make the division easier or by using powers of 10 to remove or move the decimal point.

eg $65 \div 0.25 = 65 \times 4 \div 1 = 260$.

eg $65.25 \div 5 = 130.5 \div 10 = 13.05$.

M6. Decimals 2: rounding (decimal place, significant figure) and standard form

a) Decimal place

For example, multiply 1.725 by 5 and give your answer to two decimal places (2 dp). Answer: $1.725 \times 5 = 8.625 = 8.63$ to 2 dp. Method: if the *number to the right* of the decimal place you are rounding to is 5 *or above*, then you increase the number in the decimal place by one; if it is less than 5 it remains the same. So $4.8573 = 4.857$ to 3 dp, 4.86 to 2 dp, 4.9 to 1 dp, 5.0 to 0 dp; rounding to 0 dp = rounding to the nearest whole number:

12.49 to the nearest whole number is 12 (round down);

12.50 to the nearest whole number is 13 (round up).

b) Significant figures

For example, multiply 1.725 by 5 and give your answer to two significant figures (2 sf). Answer: $1.725 \times 5 = 8.625 = 8.6$ to 2 sf. Method: similar to decimal place in that you look at the number to the right of the significant figure you are rounding to, but start from the *left-most non-zero term* (not from the decimal point). So $4.8573 = 4.857$ to 4 sf, 4.86 to 3 sf, 4.9 to 2 sf and 5.0 to 1 sf.

Any number can be rounded using significant figures: for example, $125\,890 = 130\,000$ to 2 sf; $0.003759 = 0.0038$ to 2 sf (leading zeros are not significant). Significant figures and decimal place may or may not be the same, for example: 2.916 is 2.92 to 2 dp and 2 sf; $0.02916 = 0.03$ to 2 dp, but 0.029 to 2 sf.

c) Standard form (scientific notation)

For example, 125 890 in standard form is 1.25890×10^5. Method: use powers of 10 so that only one digit comes in front of the decimal point. The following show correct and incorrect use:

$37\,500 = 3.75 \times 10^4$ in standard form.
$37\,500 = 375 \times 10^2$ true but this is not in standard form.
$0.00249 = 2.49 \times 10^{-3}$ in standard form.
$0.00249 = 0.249 \times 10^{-2}$ true but this is not in standard form.
$37\,500.00249 = 3.750000249 \times 10^4$ in standard form.
With rounding $= 3.75000025 \times 10^4$ to 9 sf; 3.7500×10^4 to 5 sf;
3.750×10^4 to 4 sf; 3.75×10^4 to 3 sf; 3.8×10^4 to 2 sf.

M7. Per cent (%)

a) Percentages

Percentages can be expressed as fractions with denominators of 100 or as decimals by moving the decimal point of the numerator two places to the left.

eg $75\% = \dfrac{75}{100} = \dfrac{15}{20} = \dfrac{3}{4}$ or $\dfrac{75.0}{100} = 0.75$

To work out a percentage figure you multiply by the percent expressed either as a fraction or as a decimal; eg 30 per cent of 120:

$$\frac{30}{100} = \frac{3}{10}; \frac{3}{10} \times 120 = 3 \times 12 = 36 \text{ or}$$

$30\% = 30 \div 100 = 0.3; 0.3 \times 120 = 3 \times 12 = 36.$

To convert any number to a percent, multiply it by 100%:

For example, $0.3 = 0.3 \times 100 = 30\%; 1.5 \times 100 = 150\%; 1/5 \times 100 = 20\%.$

Alternatively, to convert a less obvious fraction to a percent (or a decimal), express the denominator as a factor of 100.

$$\text{eg } \frac{11}{25} = \frac{11 \times 4}{25 \times 4} = \frac{44}{100} = 0.44 = 44\%$$

b) Percentage change

$$\text{Percentage change} = \frac{\text{change in value}}{\text{original value}} \times 100\%$$

Example: a car accelerates from 40 mph to 60 mph. What is the percentage increase in speed?

$$\frac{60 - 40}{40} \times 100\% = \frac{20}{40} \times 100\% = 0.5 \times 100\% = 50\% \text{ increase}$$

Example: A car brakes from 60 mph to 40 mph. What is the percentage decrease in speed?

$$\frac{60 - 40}{60} \times 100\% = \frac{20}{60} \times 100\% = \frac{1}{3} \times 100\% = 33.3\% \text{ decrease}$$

Use the original or initial value as the denominator with change.
This could also be expressed as a formula, using the symbol delta (Δ) for change and O as the original to give $\Delta/O \times 100$ = percentage change (Δ/O will give the percentage as a decimal figure).

M8. Time and clocks

a) Analogue/digital clocks

Analogue/digital clocks convert from the 12-hour clock to the 24-hour clock by re-writing the time as a four-digit number and adding 12 hours to all pm times.

For example: 8.30 am = 08:30 (oh eight-thirty hours).
10.55 pm = 10.55 + 12 hrs = 22:55 (twenty-two fifty-five hours).

Fractional parts of an hour are converted to minutes by multiplying the fraction (or its decimal) by 60 minutes:
1/4 hr = 0.25 × 60 = 15 min; 1/10 hr = 0.1 × 60 = 6 min.

You can add or subtract times as follows:
15:45 + 1 hr 50 min = 15:45 + 2 hr − 10 min = 17:35.
21:35 − 55 min = 21:35 − 1 hr + 5 min = 20:40.

Candidates should recognize the following conversions:

1 week (7 days) = 168 hours; 1 day (24 hours) = 1440 minutes.
1 hour (60 minutes) = 3600 seconds. Leap year (÷ 4) = 366 days.
eg 1.5 hr ÷ 5 = 0.3 hrs = 0.3 × 60 min = 3 × 6 min = 18 min.
eg 1 hr ÷ 100 = 1 × 60 × 60 ÷ 100 = 1 × 6 × 6 = 36 sec.

b) Clock hands questions

Wear a wrist watch if it helps!
Hour-hand rotation = 360° ÷ 12 hours = 30° per hour.
Minute-hand rotation = 360° ÷ 60 minutes = 6° per minute.
Angle between the hands: 90° at 15:00 and 21:00; 180° at 18:00.

i) **For all times when the minute hand points exactly to an hour** the angle between the hands is approximately given by:

(hr shown by hour hand − hr shown by minute hand) × 30°

and precisely by the figure given in i) plus min ÷ 60 × 30°, ie min ÷ 2° (the extra distance moved by the hour hand for the fraction of the hr).
For example, at 08:20 the angle between the hands is approx (8−4) × 30° = 120° and exactly 120° + 20 ÷ 2° = 130° (the hour hand has moved on an additional 1/3 hr (10°) in 20 minutes).

ii) **For all times when the minute hand does not point to a full hour** it can be shown that the angle between the hands is given by:

$(30° × hr – 6° × min) + min ÷ 2°$

For example, at 08:25 the angle between the hands = $(30° × 8 – 6° × 25) + 12.5° = 90° + 12.5° = 102.5°$ exactly.

M9. Areas, perimeters, volumes and surface area

a) Areas

- Square of side length $a = a × a = a^2$.

- Rectangle/parallelogram: base (b) × height $(h) = b × h$.

- Triangle: 1/2 base × vertical height = $1/2\ bh$.

- Trapezium: 'half the sum of the parallel sides × distance between them': ie ½ $(a + b)d$.

- Circle of radius r, diameter D: πr^2 (pi r squared) or as $D = 2r$: $\pi D^2/4$.

- Sector of a circle: $\pi D^2/4$ × sector angle ÷ 360.

- Cylinder of base radius r and height h: $\pi r^2 h$; sphere: $4\pi r^2$.

- Border = area of outer shape – area of inner shape.

b) Perimeters

The perimeter is the distance all the way around the outside of the shape. Examples are: square = 4 × length of side; rectangle = 2 × length × breadth; circumference of a circle $C = 2\pi r = \pi D$; perimeter of a sector = $(\pi D$ × sector angle ÷ 360) + $r + r$.

c) Volumes of solids

- Cube of side length $a = a × a × a = a^3$.

- For any uniform prism: area of cross-section × the length (or base × height × length).

- For a sphere: $4/3\ \pi r^3$.

- For a cone or pyramid: 1/3 area of base × height.

d) Surface area

This is total amount of exposed area.

- Cube = $6a^2$.
- Rectangular prism, base b, length l, height h: $2(bh + lh + bl)$.
- Hollow cylinder: circumference × height = $2\pi rh$.
- Solid cylinder: $2\pi rh + 2(\pi r^2)$.

e) Ratios of lengths, areas and volumes

For similar shapes, if the ratio of the side lengths is $a:b$ ('a to b') then the ratio of the areas is $a^2:b^2$ and the ratio of the volumes is $a^3:b^3$. For example, for two cubes of side lengths 4 cm and 2 cm respectively the ratio of side lengths is $4:2 = 2$, the ratio of the face areas is then $2^2 = 4$ and the ratio of the volumes is $2^3 = 8$ (check: 64 cm^3:8 cm^3).

M10. Algebra 1: substitution and re-arranging

a) Substitution

Letters are used in place of numbers (constants) to describe the 'general case' of something; x and y (variables) are the most common letters used in algebra. For example, substitute $x = 6$ and $y = 9$ in $x^2 - 3y + 3$; $36 - 27 + 3 = 12$.

b) Expanding brackets

i) **Any 'term' outside a bracket** multiplies each of the terms inside the bracket, moving from left to right: $5(y - 3z) = 5 \times y + 5 \times -3z = 5y - 15z$. Similarly: $-2y(7 - 4x + z) = -14y + 8xy - 2yz$.

ii) **Pair of brackets, four terms:** $(a + b)(c + d) = ac + bc + ad + bd$ (multiply everything in the second brackets by everything in the first: 'FOIL': Firsts (ac), Insides (bc), Outsides (ad), Lasts (bd)).

c) Re-arranging

Terms containing the letter you want are moved to one side of the equation (eg the left-hand side).

i) **Linear equations:** eg $x = y + z$ can be re-arranged to make y the subject by subtracting z from both sides of the equation: *leaves y on its own*: $x - z = y + z - z$ giving $x - z = y$; ie $y = x - z$.

For example, find x if $4x + y = z$:
Step 1: subtract y from both sides to give $4x + y - y = z - y$ so $4x = z - y$;
Step 2: divide both sides by 4.

$$\frac{4x}{4} = \frac{z - y}{4} \text{ then } x = \frac{z - y}{4}$$

Examples of linear equations (formulae) are temperature conversions (°C to °F) and electricity charges; for example, to convert temperature from °F to °C: $F = 9/5\ C + 32$.

To make °C the subject:

Step 1: subtract 32 from both sides to give: $F - 32 = 9/5\ C + 0$.
Step 2: multiply both sides by 5/9 to give $5/9(F - 32) = 5/9 \times 9/5\ C$;
$5/9\ (F - 32) = 1 \times C$, ie $C = 5/9\ (F - 32)$.

ii) **Equations with fractions:** eg $y = \dfrac{x + 3}{5} - \dfrac{x}{2}$; multiply by the lowest common denominator (LCD = 10) to remove the fractions, giving $10y = 2(x + 3) - 5x$, before expanding the brackets and collecting like terms: $10y = 6 - 3x$. If the denominators contain variables you can multiply them to find a common denominator.

iii) **Equations with square-root signs:** square both sides if the letter you want is inside the square-root sign.

M11. Algebra 2: simultaneous and quadratic equations

a) Factorizing

This is the reverse of expanding the brackets (M10b).

i) **'Difference of two squares'**: $x^2 - y^2 = (x + y)(x - y)$;
$16a^2 - 9b^2 = (4a)^2 - (3b)^2 = (4a + 3b)(4a - 3b)$.

ii) **'Trinomial'**: $x^2 + bx + c$ factorize by finding two numbers that when added together equal b and multiplied together equal c. For example, $x^2 + 5x + 6$; $(x\ \ )(x\ \ )$; find a pair of factors of 6 (1 and 6; 2 and 3 are the choices) that when multiplied give +6 and when added give +5, ie 2 and 3: $(x + 2)(x + 3)$.

Example: $x^2 - x - 12$; $(x\ \ )(x\ \ )$; find a pair of factors of –12 that when multiplied give –12 and when added give –1 (use trial and error on factors 1, 2, 3, 4, 6, 12 (one +, the other –) to find the solutions 3 and –4, ie $(x + 3)(x - 4)$.

In a 'perfect square' the b-term is twice the size of that inside the bracket.
For example, $x^2 + 10x + 25 = (x + 5)^2$; solve $x^2 + 6x + 2 = 0$; $(x + 3)^2 - 7 = 0$; $x + 3 = \sqrt{7}$, giving $x = -3 +/- \sqrt{7}$

b) Simultaneous equations

Expand brackets; collect x and y terms on the left-hand side; multiply by factors to make coefficients of one term equal (eg y) then add or subtract to eliminate one term (y) and solve for the other (x).
For example, 1) $5x = 3y + 33$; 2) $3(4x - y) = 12 - 7y$; solve for x and y:

Expand brackets and collect x and y terms on the left-hand side:
1) $5x - 3y = 33$;
2) $12x + 4y = 12$.

Make the coefficients of y the same in each equation, as follows:
1) × 4 gives $20x - 12y = 132$; 2) × 3 gives $36x + 12y = 36$.

Add 1) and 2): $56x = 168$ so $x = 3$; $x = 3$ in 1) gives $3y = 15 - 33$, so $y = -6$.

c) Quadratic equations: $x^2 + bx + c = 0$

i) **Solve with factors** (see also a) ii above) eg $x^2 - 6x + 5 = 0$;
$(x \quad)(x \quad)$; $(x - 5)(x - 1)$; so either $x - 5 = 0$ or $x - 1 = 0$, giving $x = 5$ or 1 as the solutions for x ('the roots').

ii) **For 'non-factorizing' quadratic equations** solve for a, b and c in the expression $ax^2 + bx + c = 0$ using the general solution:

$$x = \frac{-b \pm \sqrt{b^2 - 4ac}}{2a}$$

Using the coefficients (a, b, c) from $x^2 - 6x + 5 = 0$ gives $a = 1$, $b = -6$ and $c = 5$; so $x = (6 \pm \sqrt{36 - 20}) \div 2$; therefore $x = (6 + \sqrt{16}) \div 2$ or $x = (6 - \sqrt{16}) \div 2$; giving $x = (10) \div 2$ or $x = (2) \div 2$; ie $x = 5$ or 1 as before (example only; use if there are no obvious factors).

M12. Averages: mean, median, mode; weighted

a) Averages

i) Mean: the total of the numbers divided by the number of numbers.

ii) Median: the middle number in a group of numbers that have been ranked in numerical order from lowest to highest.

iii) Mode: the value that occurs most frequently.

For example, the weights in kilograms of seven students were as follows:
60 kg, 73 kg, 66 kg, 69 kg, 57 kg, 60 kg, 71 kg.

i) Mean = 456 kg ÷ 7 = 65.1 kg.

ii) Median: 57, 60, 60, **66**, 69, 71, 73; the middle number is 66.

　　If there is an even number of numbers then there is no 'middle value' as such, so you need to calculate the mean of the two middle numbers. To find the middle of a large group of numbers you add 1 to the number of numbers (n) and divide by 2; ie $(n + 1) \div 2$. Take for example 100 numbers: $(n + 1) \div 2 = (100 + 1) \div 2 = 50.5$ so the median is the mean of the 50th and 51st numbers.

iii) Mode = 60 because it occurs the most frequently (twice). If two values occur with equal frequency then the group is bi-modal. If more than two numbers are equally popular then the mode is not used for expressing the average value.

iv)   Range = maximum minus the minimum: 73 − 60 = 13 kg.

b) Weighted average

Some exam results count more than others towards the final result, as with university degree classifications. Example: a ratio of 1:3 for the 4th-year marks to the 5th-year marks; ie 4th year = 25 per cent; 5th year = 75 per cent. Overall percentage is given by Yr4 × 25 per cent + Yr5 × 75 per cent. Suppose that a student scores 120 out of 200 in year 4 and 240 out of 300 in Year 5. If the tests are weighted 25 per cent for Year 4 and 75 per cent for Year 5, what is the overall percentage mark?

Yr 4: 120/200 × 100% = 60%; Yr 5: 240/300 × 100% = 80%.
Now apply the weighting: overall % = 60 × 25% + 80 × 75% = 15 + 60 = 75%.

General case: **multiply each percentage mark by its percentage weight and add the results together.**

M13. Pie and bar charts, line and scatter graphs, tables

a) Pie charts

These display the relative sizes of component parts. Full circle (360°) = 100% of the data; 180° = one-half (50%), 120° = one-third (33.3%), 90° = one-quarter (25%). Each degree = 1/360th of the total quantity. Multiplying the total by the fraction/percentage gives the number for the sector. Always check for a key or subheading, especially with twin charts.

b) Bar charts (graphs)

These compare different categories of data, for example A-level subjects, or school results in different years. The bars can be drawn vertically or horizontally and the height (or length) of each bar corresponds to the size of the data. In stacked (compound) bar charts the bars are split into two or more lengths that represent different data sets, making it easier to compare the data than when bars are placed side by side. In a histogram the data are grouped into class intervals along the x-axis, for example 10–19, 20–29, 30–39 and so on, to show the distribution of the data; the data intervals are continuous so the bars must touch. NB the *area* of the bar represents the size of the data (bars can be wider or narrower depending on the class interval, eg age 40–59 is twice as wide as 30–39).

c) Line graphs

The data (displayed in a table) are plotted as a series of points joined by straight lines. The controlling quantity (eg time) is plotted on the x-axis and the quantity it controls (eg distance travelled) is plotted on the y-axis. In multiple line graphs, two or more lines are shown together on the same axes to facilitate comparisons, for example results in physics, chemistry and biology A levels. The gradient (m) of a straight line can be found by choosing two convenient points on the line, then $y = mx + c$ where gradient (m) = change in y ÷ change in x, and c is the value of y where the line intercepts the y-axis ($x = 0$).

d) Scatter graphs

These look similar to line graphs without the line, in other words with the plotted points only. Sometimes a 'line of best fit' is drawn through all of the points (not point to point). This 'regression line' can be judged by eye (and extrapolated) or it can be calculated. The line identifies the extent of any relationship (*correlation*) between the x and y values. In a strong correlation the points lie close to a straight line; x and y increase (*positive correlation*) or decrease (*negative correlation*) in proportion to each other. In a weak correlation the points are not close to the line; a state of no correlation exists if the points appear to be randomly distributed (no line can be drawn).

e) Tables

Read along a column and down a row to locate the data; most tables will have several columns and several rows. Data in a table may be reflected in a chart.

M14. Cumulative frequency, box and whisker plots

a) Cumulative frequency graphs

These are 'S'-shaped graphs showing, for example, how many candidates achieved a particular mark and below. The running total of frequencies (not the actual frequency) is plotted against the data values.

i) **Median:** the *x* value of the middle data value (eg marks score) located halfway up the cumulative frequency curve (axis), ie 50% cumulative frequency (50th percentile). Half of the data fall below the *x*-value at this point on the curve and half lie above it. Percentiles divide the data into 100 equal parts.

ii) **Upper quartile** (75th percentile): three-quarters of the data fall below the *x*-value at this point on the curve and one-quarter of the data are above it (ie it shows where the top 25% lie).

iii) **Lower quartile** (25th percentile): one-quarter of the data fall below the *x*-value at this point on the curve and three-quarters of the data are above it (ie it shows where the bottom 25% lie).

iv) **Inter-quartile range** (75th percentile minus 25th percentile): shows where the middle 50% of the data lie.

b) Box and whisker plots

These are derived from cumulative frequency graphs and display several key pieces of statistical information. Two boxes and two whiskers split the data into four quarters, as shown in the figure below.

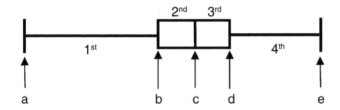

a: the lowest data value (end of whisker);
b: the lower quartile at the 25th percentile;
c: the median at the 50th percentile;
d: the upper quartile at the 75th percentile;
e: highest value (end of whisker);
d–b: the inter-quartile range (half the results lie here);
e–a: the range (end of one whisker to the end of the other).

M15. Geometry 1: angles and lines, triangles, other shapes

a) Angles and lines

i)   Where two lines intersect, the opposite angles are equal.

ii) Where a line intersects two parallel lines the corresponding angles are equal; the interior alternate angles are equal; the exterior alternate angles are equal.

iii) Angles on a straight line add up to 180°.

iv) Angles around a point add up to 360°.

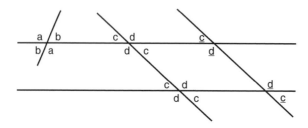

$a + b = 180°$; $c + d = 180°$; $c + d + c + d = 360°$; exterior alternate angles ($\underline{c}$) are equal; interior alternate angles ($\underline{d}$) are equal.

b) Triangles

i)   The three interior angles of any triangle add up to 180°.

ii) Scalene: all three sides are of different length.

iii) Equilateral: all sides are of equal length; all angles are equal to 60°.

iv) Isosceles: opposite sides of equal length and two angles equal.

v)   Right angle: one angle is 90°.

c) Other shapes

i) **For any regular quadrilateral** (square, rectangle, parallelogram, rhombus, trapezium, kite) and irregular quadrilaterals (any four-sided shape other than those described above): the four interior angles add up to 360°.

ii) **For any shape with _n_ sides:** the sum of the interior angles is given by $(180n - 360)°$, ie $180(n - 2)°$; for a regular polygon having all sides the same length (eg pentagon, hexagon, heptagon, octagon) each interior angle equals $180(n - 2)° \div n$.

For example, in a regular octagon: each interior angle = $180(8 - 2)° ÷ 8 = 1080 ÷ 8 = 135°$.

M16. Geometry 2: Pythagoras and trigonometric functions

a) Pythagoras' theorem for any right-angled triangle

Opposite^2 + adjacent^2 = hypotenuse^2 (longest side).

In other words, if you know the length of two sides you can use Pythagoras to find the third side. The six smallest Pythagorean triples (sides with whole numbers) are (3,4,5), (5,12,13), (6,8,10), (9,12,15), (8,15,17), (7,24,25); for instance, $3^2 + 4^2 = 5^2$ (ie a 3,4,5 triangle). Four of the above triples are primitives and two are non-primitives (6,8,10), (9,12,15). All Pythagorean triples are *multiples* of one of the primitives, for example (3,4,5) × 2 = (6,8,10); × 3 = (9,12,15); × 4 = (12,16,20); (7,24,25) × 2 = (14,48,50).

b) Sin, cosine and tan: (angle depends on ratio of side lengths)

i) **Right-angled triangles:**
sin = opposite ÷ hypotenuse; cos = adjacent ÷ hypotenuse;
tan = opposite ÷ adjacent. 'SOH…CAH…TOA'.
eg for a 6,8,10 triangle we have:

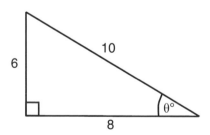

sin θ = 6/10 = 0.6; cos θ = 8/10 = 0.8; tan θ = 6/8 = 0.75.
Inverse functions θ = sin^{-1} 0.6 = cos^{-1} 0.8 = tan^{-1} 0.75.

ii) **Non-right-angled triangles:** when a is the side opposite angle A, b is the side opposite angle B and c is opposite angle C then (when three pieces of data are known).

Sine law: a ÷ sin A = b ÷ sin B = c ÷ sin C (used when at least one angle and its opposite side are known (eg A and a), plus one more side or one more angle.
Cosine law: $a^2 = b^2 + c^2 - 2bc \cos A$ (used when all three side-lengths are known or two sides and the angle between them).

iii) **Angles greater than 90°**, sin x = sin (180 − x); −cos x = cos (180 − x); for example, x = 120°; sin 120 = sin 60; −cos 120 = cos 60.
Sine wave: graph of y = sin x; amplitude = 1 (y-axis), period (x-axis) = 360° (2π); for example, graph of y = 10 sin x; amplitude = 10, period = 360° (2π); sine is negative for angles between 180° and 360° wave goes below the x-axis.
Cosine wave: same as sine wave only shifted to the left by 90° (π/2); cos is negative for angles between 90° and 270°; wave goes below the x-axis.

M17. Circle theorems

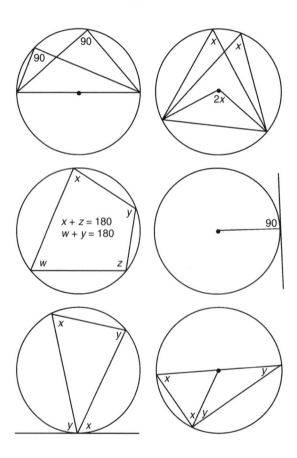

M18. Inequalities

a) Linear inequalities

For example:

i) **Solve** $x - 6 < 0$ (x minus 6 is less than 0); add 6 to both sides to give $x < 6$.

ii) **Solve** $-x^2 + 9 < 0$; subtract 9 from both sides to give:
$-x^2 < -9$ then *multiply both sides by –1 and reverse the inequality sign* ie $x^2 > 9$
so $x > 3$.

iii) **Solve** $5x - 12 > 8$ ($5x$ minus 12 is greater than 8); add 12 to both sides to give:
$5x > 20$ so $x > 4$.

iv) **Solve** $4 - 3x < 10$; subtract 4 from both sides to give $-3x < 6$;
divide both sides by –3 and reverse the inequality sign: $x > -2$.

v) **Find the range** for x in $-4 < 3x + 5 < 11$; subtract 5 from all three parts to give
$-9 < 3x < 6$; dividing by 3 gives $-3 < x < 2$.

vi) **Solve** $8 - 2x \le 5$ (8 minus $2x$ is less than or equal to 5); subtract 8 from both sides
to give $-2x \le -3$ then multiply both sides by –1 and reverse the sign to give $2x \ge 3$ so
$x \ge 1.5$.

b) Quadratic inequalities

For example: find the range of values of x for which $x^2 - 8x < -12$; add 12 to both
sides: $x^2 - 8x + 12 < 0$ then treat as a normal quadratic: $x^2 - 7x + 12 = 0$ to get the
roots, ie $(x - 2)(x - 6)$, so $x = 2$ or 6.
   To find the range of values for $x^2 - 8x + 12 < 0$, graph the data for $x^2 - 7x + 12$
$= y$ and find the range of x values for which $y < 0$. Draw the graph from $y = 0$ when
$x = 2$ or 6; $y = 12$ when $x = 0$, $(x^2 - 8x + 12 = y)$; quadratic equations form parabolic/
U-shaped curves.

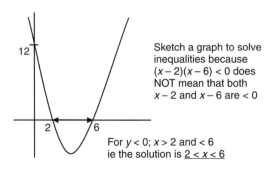

Sketch a graph to solve
inequalities because
$(x - 2)(x - 6) < 0$ does
NOT mean that both
$x - 2$ and $x - 6$ are < 0

For $y < 0$; $x > 2$ and < 6
ie the solution is $\underline{2 < x < 6}$

M19. Probability 1: basic concepts

a) Defining probability (P)

P values range from 0 to 1 and can be written as a decimal, percentage, fractions or ratio:

$0 = 0\% =$ impossible.
$0.1 = 10\%$ certainty, 1/10 or 1 in 10 chance (1:10).
$0.25 = 25\%$ certainty, 1/4 or 1 in 4 chance (1:4).
$0.5 = 50\%$ certainty, 1/2 or 1 in 2 chance (1:2).
$0.75 = 75\%$ certainty, 3/4 or 3 in 4 chance (3:4).
$1 = 100\%$ certainty.

Also: 50% certainty = 50% uncertainty ('fifty-fifty').
Similarly: 40% certainty = 60% uncertainty ('forty-sixty').

b) Equation

Probability of a given event E, $P(E)$ is given by:

$P(E) =$ number of times E occurs $\div$ total number of outcomes.

c) The 'and' rule and the 'or' rule

For independent events:

i) Probability (P) of A *and* $B = P(A) \times P(B)$; that is to say, the probability of both equals the product of the individual probabilities. For example, find the probability of throwing a 3 *and* a 4 on a dice with two successive throws: $P(A \text{ and } B) = P(A)$ $P(B) = 1/6 \times 1/6 = 1/36$.

ii) Probability (P) of A *or* $B = P(A) + P(B)$.
For example, find the probability of throwing a 6 *or* a 4 on a dice: $P(A \text{ or } B) = P(A) +$ $P(B) = 1/6 + 1/6 = 2/6 = 1/3$.

For dependent events:

iii) $P(A \text{ and } B) = P(A) \, P(B \text{ after A})$.
For example, find the probability of drawing an ace from a 52-card pack, then drawing a second ace without putting the first one back:

P(A *and* B) = P(A) P(B after A) = 4/52 × 3/51 = 1/13 × 1/17.

For example, find the probability of drawing a black card *or* a king from a 52–card pack:

P(A *or* B) = P(A) + P(B) – P(A *and* B).

P(A *or* B) = 26/52 + 2/52 –(26/52 × 2/52) = 28/52 –1/52 = 27/52.

(26 black cards and 2 black kings, ie not mutually exclusive.)

For mutually exclusive events:

iv) P(A *and* B) = P(A) × P(B) = 0; P(A *or* B) = P(A) + P(B) = 1; eg tossing a coin: probability of a head and tail together = 0; probability of a head or a tail = 1.

M20. Probability 2: tree diagrams

a) Rules

The total of the probabilities on two branches from a single point = 1; probabilities add vertically and multiply horizontally from branch to branch.

Example: A car manufacturer buys 80% (0.8) of its widgets from Firm A and the remainder from Firm B. Two % of the widgets from Firm A are defective and 5% of the widgets from Firm B are defective. If one widget is withdrawn from a mixed bag of widgets, find the probability that:

i)   The widget will be defective and made by Firm A.

ii)   The widget will be defective and made by Firm B.

iii) The widget will be defective and made by either firm.

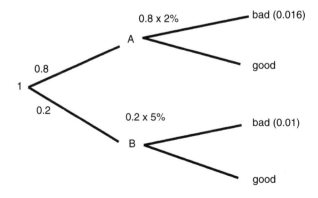

i)   0.016 (1.6%); ii) 0.01 (1%); iii) 0.016 + 0.01 = 0.026 (2.6%).

Example: 10 000 people are tested for a drug. Of these, 1% are drug users and the rest are not. For drug users there is a 1% chance of a false negative and for non-drug users there is a 1% chance of a false positive. What is the probability that a person chosen at random who tests positive is actually a drug user?

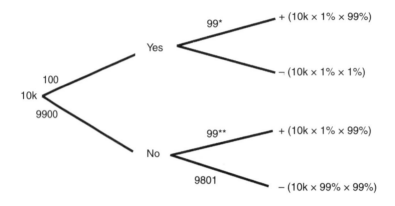

Probability $E = 99* \div (99* + 99**) = 99 \div 198 = 50$ per cent.

M21. Permutations and combinations

a) Counting principle

For example, a car is available in eight different colours, four engine sizes and three levels of trim $= 8 \times 4 \times 3 = 96$ choices.

b) Permutations

i) **Permutations for a set $n = n!$ (ie n factorial)**
(factorial $10 = 10 \times 9 \times 8 \times 7 \times 6 \times 5 \times 4 \times 3 \times 2 \times 1$).
For example, permutations of a three-letter group, A,B,C, are as follows:

ABC, ACB, BAC, BCA, CAB, CBA (the order of selection is important);
ie Permutation $P = 6 = 3 \times 2 \times 1$ (ie 3 factorial; 3!);

For a four-letter group A,B,C,D; $P = 4! = 4 \times 3 \times 2 \times 1 = 24$.

ii) **Permutations of r objects from a set $n = n! \div (n - r)!$**
For example, the number of possible permutations of any two-letter group chosen from a group of 10 letters A,B,C,D,E,F,G,H,I,J is given by: $P = 10 \div (10 - 2)! = 10! \div 8!$
$= 10 \times 9 = 90$.

c) Combinations

i) Combination for objects from a set $n = n! \div (n - k)!k!$

For example, the number of possible combinations of any two-letter group chosen from a group of 10 letters A,B,C,D,E,F,G,H,I,J (the order of selection is not important) is given by:

$C = 10! \div (10 - 2)!2! = 10! \div 8!2! = 10 \times 9 \div 2! = 45$ possible ways of choosing two letters from 10.

d) Combinations vs permutations

Example: in eight-ball pool there are eight balls numbered from 1 to 8. These are placed in a sack and three balls are drawn out at random. i) How many different combinations of three balls are possible? ii) How many different permutations of three balls are possible?

i) $C = 8! \div (8 - 3)!3! = 8! \div 5!3! = 8 \times 7 \times 6 \div 3 \times 2 = 56$.
ii) $P = 8! \div (8 - 3) = 8! \div 5! = 8 \times 7 \times 6 = 336$.

For example, balls 1, 2 and 3 = one combination of balls with six possible permutations (1,2,3; 1,3,2; 2,1,3; 2,3,1; 3,1,2; 3,2,1 or 3!)

Maths review questions

Q1   (M9) If the area of the square in the figure below is 4 cm², what is the area of the shaded region?

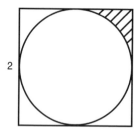

2

    A. $4 - \pi$
    B. $2 - \pi$
    C. $1 - 0.5\pi$
    D. $1 - 0.25\pi$
    E. 0.75π

Answer [   ]

Q2   (M16) What is the area of the square?

A   D

10 cm

B   C

    A. 100 cm²
    B. $\sqrt{200}$ cm²
    C. $\sqrt{50}$ cm²
    D. $\sqrt{150}$ cm²
    E. 50 cm²

Answer [   ]

Q3   (M9, 16) ABC is an equilateral triangle of side x. What is its area?

A. $x^2(3/4)$
B. $\sqrt{3}(x^2/4)$
C. $2x(\sqrt{3})$
D. $10\sqrt{3}$
E. $3x/4$

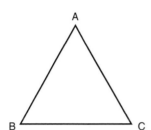

(hint: split base in two)

Answer ☐

Q4   (M16) What is the length of h in the triangle shown below?

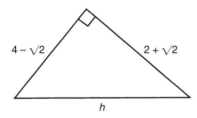

A. $2\sqrt{(6-\sqrt{2})}$
B. $6(4-\sqrt{2})$
C. $6\sqrt{2}$
D. $2(6-\sqrt{2})$
E. $2\sqrt{(4-\sqrt{2})}$

Answer ☐

Q5   (M15) The area of the shape ABCD is 60 cm². What is its perimeter?

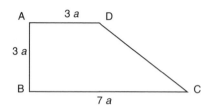

A. 30 cm
B. 32 cm
C. 34 cm
D. 36 cm
E. 38 cm

Answer

Q6   (M17) What is the length of the arc AB if the circle has a diameter of 10 cm?

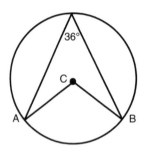

A. 2π cm
B. 3π cm
C. 4π cm
D. 6π cm

(hint: circle theorem)

Answer

Q7   (M2) Calculate $[6^{2/3}]^6 + [10^{4/5}]^5$.

A. 1.75×10^{11}
B. 1.296×10^8
C. 1.1296×10^4
D. 1.6×10^5

Answer

Q8   (M2) Calculate $\dfrac{9 \times 2^{15} - 6 \times 8^5}{3 \times 8^5}$

Answer

Q9   (M10, 11) Find x if $(5x - 2)^2 = 4$.

Answer

Q10   (M10, 11) If $(2x)^8 = (2x + 3)^4$, what is one possible value of x?

A. 1/4
B. 1/3
C. 4/3
D. 3/2

Answer

Q11   (M10, 11) A purse contains £5.70 in a mixture of 50p and 20p coins. If there are 15 coins in total, how many of these are 20p coins?

Answer

Q12   (M9, 11) Cubes A, B and C fit snugly into cube D. The volume of cube A is eight times that of cube B and the volume of cube C is one-eighth that of cube B. If the volume of cube D is 1000 cm³, what is the side-length of cube A?

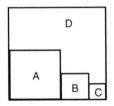

A. $2^2/_6$
B. $5^5/_7$
C. $4^6/_7$
D. $6^3/_7$

Answer

Q13 (M11) In a quadratic equation, the sum of the roots is 0 and the product of the roots is −16. What is the equation?

A. $x^2 + 8 = 0$
B. $x^2 − 8 = 0$
C. $x^2 + 16 = 0$
D. $x^2 − 16 = 0$

Answer [   ]

Q14 (M19ciii) You are dealt two cards from a shuffled pack of 52 playing cards. What is the probability that the first card will be a spade and the second card will be a spade?

A. 1:15
B. 1:16
C. 1:17
D. 1:18

Answer [   ]

Q15 (M18) Solve the inequality $x(2x + 6) \le 8$.

A. $x = 1; x = −4$
B. $x \le 1; x \le −4$
C. $4 \le x \le −1$
D. $−4 \le x \le 1$

Answer [   ]

Q16 (M10) If $a = \dfrac{y - b}{y - c}$, express y in terms of a and b.

A. $(ac − b)/(a − 1)$
B. $(a − 1)/(ac − b)$
C. $(b − ac)/(a − 1)$
D. $(ac + b)/(a − 1)$

Answer [   ]

Q17 (M16biii) If a cosine graph is 90° out of phase with the sine graph shown below, and the cosine of 0° = 1, which of the following statements must be true?

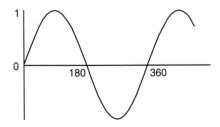

A. sin 90 = cos 180
B. sin 0 = cos 180
C. sin 180 = cos 360
D. sin 90 = – cos 90
E. sin 270 = cos 180

(hint: draw cos)

Answer [   ]

CHAPTER 3

Physics review

P1.   Measurements and prefixes
P2.   Conventions for units, symbols and numbers
P3.   SI base units for length, volume, mass
P4.   Equations of motion
P5.   Graphs of motion
P6.   Projectile motion
P7.   Force and motion (Newton)
P8.   Force, work, power and energy
P9.   Universal gravitation, satellites and escape velocity
P10. Force, momentum and impulse
P11. Force, stress and strain
P12. Moments, mechanical advantage, levers and pulleys
P13. Pressure, buoyancy and flow
P14. Gas laws
P15. Heat and energy
P16. Waves (light and sound)
P17. Electrostatics, capacitance and electricity
P18. Kirchhoff's circuit laws, resistors and capacitors
P19. Electromagnetism and electromagnetic induction
P20. Radioactive decay
      Physics review questions

P1. Measurements and prefixes

a) The SI system

There are seven base units in the SI system: length in metres (m), mass in kilograms (kg), time in seconds (s), electric current in amperes (A), temperature in kelvins (K), luminous intensity in candelas (cd) and amount of substance in moles (mol). The remaining SI units are derived from combinations of these base units. For example:

joules (J) $= kg\ m^2\ s^{-2}$;
volts (V) $= kg\ m^2\ s^{-3}\ A^{-1}$.

Base units help to reveal links between derived units; in the above examples the $kg\ m^2$ terms can be cancelled to give:

$J/V = A\ s$, so $J = V\ A\ s$;
and ampere second $=$ coulomb (C).
Thus $J = V\ C$ (joules $=$ volts $\times$ coulombs)

b) SI prefixes

The following SI prefixes describe orders of magnitude ranging from 10^{-12} to 10^{+12} and most are in steps of 1000.

Factor	Name	Symbol	Example
10^{-12}	pico	p	picofarad (pF)
10^{-9}	nano	n	nanometre (nm)
10^{-6}	micro	μ	microgram (μg)
10^{-3}	milli	m	milligram (mg)
10^{-2}	centi	c	centimetre (cm)
10^{-1}	deci	d	decilitre (dl)
10^{+3}	kilo	k	kilonewton (kN)
10^{+6}	mega	M	megapascal (MPa)
10^{+9}	giga	G	gigajoule (GJ)
10^{+12}	tera	T	terawatts (TW)

P2. Conventions for units, symbols and numbers

Use the following conventions when writing SI units, symbols and numbers:

a)   Choose units that limit the use of decimals, fractions or numbers greater than 1000. For example, use 500 micrograms NOT 0.5 mg; 1.5 mg NOT 1500 micrograms; avoid Greek letters and write out microgram in full (on prescriptions) to avoid confusion with mg.

b)   Leave a space between the number and the unit and avoid plurals (s); for example, 25 mg NOT 25mg or 25 mgs; 2.5 L NOT 2.5L.

c)   With the exception of the litre (L), the symbols for units should be in lower-case letters unless the unit is named after an individual. For example, metre (m); second (s); kilometre (km); but volts (V); newtons (N); watts (W); joules (J); kelvins (K).

d)   A forward slash or a negative exponent can be used to separate the top unit from any unit it is divided by, but use only exponents if more than one slash is required. For example, g/cm^3 or $g\ cm^{-3}$; m/s^2 or $m\ s^{-2}$ but for clarity $kg/m/s^2$ should be written as $kg\ m^{-1}\ s^{-2}$.

e)   Use gaps to break up large numbers into groups of three digits; a comma is non-standard because it is a decimal separator in some European countries. No gap is required with four-digit numbers, though you may use one if you wish.

For example, 1 275 000; 1,275,000 is non-standard (but frequently used); 0.259 75 NOT 0.259,75; 5002 (or 5 002) but NOT 5,002.

f)   Do not use a multiplication sign between units; use a space or a raised dot. For example, newton metre: N m (or N·m), NOT N × m.

P3. SI base units for length, volume, mass

a) Length

1 metre (m) = 100 centimetres (cm).
1 kilometre (km) = 1000 metres (m).
1 centimetre = 10 mm (mm).
1 mm = 1000 micrometres (1000 microns (non-SI)).
1 micrometre (μm) = 0.001 mm = 0.000 001 metres (10^{-6} m).
1 nanometre = 10^{-9} m (and 1 ångström (non-SI) = 0.1 nanometre).

b) Mass

1 kilogram (kg) = 1000 grams (g).
1 gram (g) = 1000 milligrams (mg).
1 milligram (mg) = 1000 micrograms.
1 metric ton (t) = 1000 kg = 1 megagram (Mg).

c) Volume

1 litre (L or l) = 1000 millilitres (mL).
1 decilitre (dL) = 0.1 L = 100 mL.
1 centilitre (cL) = 0.01 l = 10 mL.
1 millilitre (mL) = 0.001 litre.
1 ml = 1 cm^3 and 1 L = 1000 cm^3.
1 microlitre (μL) = 0.001 mL = 0.000 001 l (10^{-6} mL) .
1 cubic metre (m^3) = 1000 L.
1 cubic decimetre (dm^3) = 1 litre.

d) Density

Density (ρ) = mass per unit volume (g cm^{-3} or kg m^{-3}); 1 g cm^{-3} = 1000 kg m^{-3}.
Relative density (specific gravity) = density relative to water (no units). The density of water can be taken as 1 g cm^{-3} (= 1 kg L^{-3} = 1 t m^{-3}).

P4. Equations of motion

a) Speed is a scalar quantity measured in metres per second.

Average speed = distance ÷ time taken (m s^{-1}); distance = speed × time.

b) Velocity is a vector; it measures speed in a given direction.

Average velocity = net displacement ÷ time taken (m s^{-1}).
Zero net displacement = zero average velocity.
For example, a car travels 10 km north and then 10 km south at an average speed of 50 kilometres per hour. Net displacement = 0 (10 and –10); average velocity = 0.
(NB distance travelled = 20 km; displacement = 0 km.)
With uniform (constant) velocity the magnitude of the speed and the direction of motion remain constant.

c) Acceleration is a vector that measures change in velocity per second; the units are metres per second per second (ie metres per second squared ($m\ s^{-2}$)).

acceleration (a) = change in velocity (v in $m\ s^{-1}$) ÷ time taken ($\times s^{-1}$)
= ($v - u$)/t (final velocity v; initial velocity u)
= v/t (when $u = 0$, ie 'from a standing start').

d) There are three more equations that describe motion under uniform (constant) acceleration:

$v = u + at$;
$v^2 = u^2 + 2as$;
$s = ut + 1/2at^2$;
where s = distance travelled in time t.

e) In circular motion the direction is continually changing so acceleration is taking place; this *centripetal acceleration* is towards the centre of the circle and is given by: $a = v^2/r$ (where r = radius); for one revolution, distance = circumference = $2\pi r$ so $2\pi r = vT$ (distance = velocity × time) and $T = 2\pi r/v$ (where T = time for one revolution, or the 'period').

P5. Graphs of motion

a) Distance versus time graphs

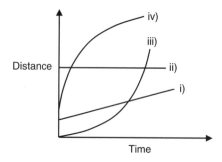

i) Constant velocity: *slope of the line = velocity*.

ii) Zero velocity (stationary/at rest; no slope).

iii) Increasing velocity = positive acceleration (becoming steeper).

iv) Decreasing velocity = negative acceleration (becoming less steep), for example, when braking and coming to a halt (line eventually horizontal).

b) *Velocity versus time graphs*

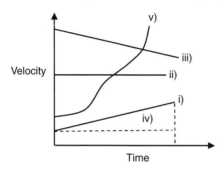

i)   Increasing velocity = *slope of line* = *uniform (constant) acceleration*.

ii)   Uniform velocity = constant speed.

iii) Decreasing velocity = uniform deceleration.

iv)   Distance travelled = area under the graph (triangle + rectangle).

v)   Non-uniform velocity (count full and half squares to calculate area).

P6. Projectile motion

a)   Substitute g (acceleration due to gravity) for a, and h (height) for s in the equations of motion:

$v = u + gt$ $v^2 = u^2 + 2gh$ $h = ut + 1/2gt^2$.

b)   Time: for an object thrown vertically upwards, the time to reach the highest point (u known) is given by $v = u + at$ and $v = 0$ at the highest point so $0 = u - gt$, giving $t = u/g$. The object takes the same amount of time to return to the ground and arrives at the same speed that it left, so total flight time = $2u/g$.

c)   Height: for an object dropped vertically from a cliff or down a well (t known, $u = 0$), calculate the height (h) from $h = 1/2gt^2$ or $5gt^2$ (take $g = -10$ m s^{-2}).

d)   Height: for an object thrown vertically upwards from the ground (u known), calculate the maximum height (h) from $v^2 = u^2 + 2gh$ with $v = 0$ at the highest point, so $h = u^2/2g$ or $u^2/20$ ($g = -10$ m s^{-2}; deceleration).

e)   Range: for an object thrown horizontally from a cliff known, treat the horizontal motion (x-direction) and the vertical motion (y-direction) separately. Calculate the range (x) from $x = vt$ where v is the horizontal velocity, and t is the time in flight; t can be calculated from the drop height: $h = 1/2\,gt^2$ so $t = \sqrt{(2h/g)}$.

f)   (Unlikely to be tested) For projectiles fired at an angle of θ to the horizontal, the maximum range (x) occurs when $\theta = 45°$; then the height and range;

h is given by: $(u^2 \sin^2\theta)/2g$ ie $u^2/4g$ at 45° (half that of h at 90°);

x is given by: $(u^2 \sin 2\theta)/g$ ie u^2/g at 45° (twice h at 90°).

For example, a projectile is fired vertically and reaches a height of 2000 m.

b) Time to the highest point given by: $h = 0.5gt^2$; $t = \sqrt{(2h/g)}$.

$t = \sqrt{(4000/g)} = \sqrt{(400)} = 20$ s; time of flight 20 s × 2 = 40 s.

b) Initial velocity: from $t = u/g$, $u = tg = 200$ m s^{-1}.

f) Fired at 45° to the horizontal the projectile would achieve a height of 1000 m and a range of 4000 m (ignoring air resistance).

P7. Force and motion (Newton)

a)   Newton's first law: a body remains stationary or in uniform motion unless acted on by a force (such as friction).

b)   Newton's second law: a force causes an acceleration: $F = ma$ where F is in newtons, m in kilograms and a in m s^{-2}; a force of one newton gives an acceleration of one metre per second squared to a mass of one kilogram.

c)   Acceleration due to gravity is 9.81 m s^{-2} or ≈ 10 m s^{-2} so the force on a mass of 1 kg, experienced as weight (W), is:

$W = mg \approx 1 \times 10$ N ie 1 kg weight ≈ 10 N (downwards).

d)   Circular motion: the acceleration towards the centre is given by $a = v^2/r$ and since $F = ma$ then $F = mv^2/r$ where r = radius of the circle.

e)   Newton's third law: action and reaction are equal; that is to say, forces come in pairs. Weight, for example, is supported by a force *normal* (perpendicular) to the surface.

f)   Friction force (tangential) necessary for an object to slide by overcoming friction is proportional to the normal force and the coefficient of friction (μ). Friction force = μ × normal force.

g)   Terminal velocity in free fall is governed by Newton's second law; it is reached when the downward force due to gravity (the weight) is balanced by the upward friction force due to air resistance (the drag); with no net force the acceleration ceases.

Net force F_{net} = Weight (W) – Drag (D).

$W - D = 0$ or $W = D$ at the terminal velocity.

The drag increases with speed and frontal area. Heavier objects reach higher terminal velocities than lighter objects of similar shape because there is more weight 'left over' after the drag.

P8. Force, work, power and energy

a)   Work done in joules (J) by a force in newtons (N) moving a distance in metres (m) is given by:

work done (J) = force × distance (N m).

Thus one joule is the work done when a force of one newton moves through a distance of one metre.

b)   Power is the rate of doing work and is measured in watts (W).

Power (W) = work done ÷ time taken (J s^{-1}).

Thus one watt is the power required to move a force of one newton through a distance of one metre in one second.

For someone of mass m (kg) to run upstairs climbing a height h (metres) in time t (s), the power required is given by:

Power (W) = force × distance ÷ time taken = mgh/t;

= force × velocity = mgv.

c)   Energy is the capacity to do work and, like work done, it is measured in joules. The law of conservation of energy states that energy can neither be created nor destroyed, only changed from one form to another; energy–mass equivalence:

$E = mc^2$.

Kinetic energy (KE) is the energy of motion.

Potential energy (PE) is stored energy: gravitational potential energy, chemical potential energy and elastic potential energy.

KE = $1/2\,mv^2$ and PE = mgh.

For falling bodies (or bodies thrown upwards) energy is conserved, so we have:
PE lost = KE gained (or if up, PE gained = KE lost).

Thus $mgh = 1/2\,mv^2$ or $1/2\,mv^2 + mgh$ = constant.

Note: PE gained or lost depends on changes in vertical height and *not on speed and path*.

P9. Universal gravitation, satellites and escape velocity

a)   Newton's law of universal gravitation states that every object in the universe attracts every other object with a force that is proportional to the product of their masses (m_1m_2) and inversely proportional to the square of separation (r^2) from centre to centre.

Thus $F = \dfrac{Gm^1 m^2}{r^2}$ where G is the universal gravitational constant.

On earth the force on an object of mass m is given by $F = mg$.

Thus $mg = \dfrac{GmM}{r^2}$ so $g = \dfrac{GM}{r^2}$ (earth of mass M, radius r).

Note that the gravitational force exerted by the earth on a body equals the gravitational force exerted by the body on the earth.

b) On leaving the surface of the earth, gravity decreases in inverse proportion to the square of the distance from the earth's centre. For a satellite of mass m orbiting the earth in uniform circular motion, $F = mv^2/r$ ($r =$ distance of satellite from the earth's centre).

Thus $= \dfrac{GmM}{r^2} = \dfrac{mv^2}{r}$ giving $v^2 = \dfrac{GM}{r}$ and $v = \sqrt{\dfrac{GM}{r}}$

c) For an object to escape the earth's gravitational field it must leave the surface with sufficient kinetic energy to overcome the force of gravity, at which point all its kinetic energy ($1/2\, mv^2$) will have been converted to potential energy (mgr).

Thus $1/2\, mv^2 = mgr = \dfrac{GmM}{r}$ giving $v^2 = \dfrac{2GM}{r}$ so $v = \sqrt{\dfrac{2GM}{r}}$

The escape velocity (v) is the speed that an unpowered rocket must be launched at to overcome the earth's gravity (neglecting air resistance); powered rockets can leave the earth's gravitational field at any speed.

You are unlikely to be tested on the formula but you could be given one to re-arrange.

P10. Force, momentum and impulse

a) Momentum of a moving object is the product of its mass and its velocity:

Momentum (p) = mass (m) × velocity (v) = mv;

and $F = ma$; $v = u + at$; ie $a = (v - u)/t$ so $F = m(v - u)/t$.

Thus Force = change in momentum ÷ time taken;

or Force × time = change in momentum = impulse.

b) Two objects collide (m_1 and m_2): the action and reaction forces are equal (Newton's third law) and as the contact times are the same, so are the changes in momentum.

In other words, total momentum before collision = total momentum after it.

c) Elastic collision (snooker balls): both the momentum and the kinetic energy are conserved:

conservation of momentum: $m_1u_1 + m_2u_2 = m_1v_1 + m_2v_2$;
conservation of KE: $1/2(m_1u_1^2 + m_2u_2^2) = 1/2 (m_1v_1^2 + m_2v_2^2)$.

d) Inelastic collision (car crash): the momentum is conserved but some of the kinetic energy is lost as heat. A typical collision involves one stationary object ($u_2 = 0$) and both objects sticking together after collision ($v_2 = v_1$), thus:

conservation of momentum with m_2 stationary before impact and both objects linked after the collision: $m_1u_1 = (m_1 + m_2) v_2$;
loss of kinetic energy: $1/2 \, m_1u_1^2 > 1/2(m_1 + m_2) v_2^2$.

e) Momentum is a vector. If two objects are moving towards each other then motion to the right should be signed as positive and motion to the left as negative ($m_1u_1 + m_2(-u_2)$). If elastic, the relative velocity before collision = relative velocity after collision: $V_1 - V_2 = U_2 - U_1$ (*signed vectors*); for example m_1 travelling east at 4 m s^{-1} with m_2 travelling west at 6 m s^{-1}: $U_2 - U_1 = -6 - (+4) = -10$ m s^{-1} ($= V_1 - V_2$).

P11. Force, stress and strain

a) Material under load (eg a suspension bridge cable): the stress is given by:

Stress = force ÷ area (N m^{-2} or pascals Pa); the units are the same as for pressure. The strain is given by:

Strain = extension ÷ length (no units).

For a given material:

Stress ÷ strain = constant = Young's modulus of material.
Thus the strain is proportional to the stress up to the elastic limit (Hooke's law). Beyond the limit of proportionality (elastic limit) the material only partially springs back when the load is removed, leaving it permanently stretched (plastic deformation).

b) Hooke's law for springs: the force exerted by a spring in tension is proportional to the distance (x) it is stretched (up to the elastic limit).

Force = $-kx$ where k is the spring constant (N m^{-1}).

Thus for a spring stretched to double its natural length, the return force will be half that of a spring stretched to four times its natural length. The work done in stretching (or compressing) a spring is equal to the product of the average force and the displacement (x) squared.
Thus work done = $1/2 \, kx^2$ = change in elastic potential energy.

If a stretched or compressed spring is released, the stored potential energy is converted into kinetic energy.

For an oscillating spring: Total energy = $1/2\ kx^2 + 1/2\ mv^2$ = constant.

P12. Moments, mechanical advantage, levers and pulleys

a) The moment (torque) of a force about a pivot is given by:

Moment of force = force × perpendicular distance from pivot.
For a lever balanced on a fulcrum (in equilibrium), the moments each side of the fulcrum are the same: $f_1d_1 = f_2d_2$.

b) Mechanical advantage (MA) = load ÷ effort;

(load = mechanical advantage × effort).
Velocity ratio = distance effort moves ÷ distance load moves;
(distance effort moves = velocity ratio × distance load moves).

c) A lever is a practical application of moments. If d_1 = 10 d_2, then a force of 1 N (f_1) will balance a load of 10 N (f_2).

Mechanical advantage (MA) = load ÷ effort = × 10 in above.
Velocity ratio = length of effort arm ÷ length resistance arm (× 10 above).
Mechanical advantage = velocity ratio (no units).

d) Classes of lever: these depend upon the relative positions of the pivot (fulcrum), the effort and the load.

1st class: fulcrum between load and effort (eg seesaw; triceps):
MA ≥ 1 (1st class can give the greatest magnification of force).
2nd class: load between fulcrum and effort (eg wheelbarrow):
MA > 1 (MA increases as the load approaches the fulcrum).
3rd class: effort between fulcrum and load (eg biceps):
MA < 1 (reduction in force = mechanical disadvantage; velocity ratio < 1 = magnification of movement).

e) Mechanical (machine) efficiency: the units for moment of force are N m, as per work done, and since $f_1d_1 = f_2d_2$ no energy is lost if 100 per cent efficient (ie no friction/heat losses), so: Efficiency = work output ÷ work input × 100 per cent. This efficiency = mechanical advantage ÷ velocity ratio × 100 per cent.

f) Pulley: Mechanical advantage = number of moving lines supporting the load.

P13. Pressure, buoyancy and flow

a) Solids: Pressure = force ÷ area (N m^{-2} or pascals Pa); the units are identical to those for stress; that is, pressure = mg ÷ A.

b) Liquids and gases: Pressure = force ÷ area = mg ÷ A where the mass m = density of fluid (ρ) × volume (area × depth h);

so Pressure = $pgAh$ ÷ A = pgh; ie pressure is proportional to the depth below the surface and the density of the fluid.

c) SI and non SI units for 1 atmosphere of pressure:

i) SI: 1 atmosphere (atm) = 1×10^5 Pa = 100 kPa = 100 kN m^{-2};
ii) non SI: 1 atm = 14.7 pounds per square inch (psi) = 760 mm mercury (Hg);
= 760 torr = 1 bar = 1000 millibars.

d) **Archimedes' principle:** a fully or partially immersed object experiences an upthrust equal to the weight of fluid displaced (and if submerged: volume object = volume displaced fluid (V_f)).

Upthrust (buoyancy) = $m_f g = \rho_f V_f g$ where ρ_f= density of fluid.
Net force on an immersed object: $m_o g - \rho_f V_f g$; to float = 0, so:
floating bodies displace their own weight of fluid.
For water ρ = 1 g cm^{-3} ie weight in grams = volume in ml.
For example, a submerged object of volume 100 ml has an upthrust of 100 grams; a 100-gram mass that floats displaces 100 ml of water; a 100-gram mass that displaces 90 ml water sinks (net wt = 10 g).

e) Fluid flow and the continuity equation: fluids can be considered to be incompressible so the volume of fluid exiting a pipe must equal the volume of fluid entering it, per unit time.

Flow rate = vol per sec (cm^3 s^{-1}) = area (cm^2) × velocity (cm s^{-1}).
Thus $A_1 V_1 = A_2 V_2$; inverse law: velocity up at narrow sections.

f) Bernoulli's equation for fluid flow (conservation of energy):
P (pipe pressure energy) + ρgh (PE; static head) + $1/2\rho v^2$ (KE) = **constant**
(velocity up at narrow cross sections = pressure down).

P14. Gas laws

a) Boyle's law: p proportional to 1/V ie pV = constant; $p_1 V_1 = p_2 V_2$.
Charles' law: V proportional to T ie V/T = constant; $V_1/T_1 = V_2/T_2$.
Gas law: p proportional to T ie p/T = constant; $p_1/T_1 = p_2/T_2$.

(T absolute: kelvin = °Celsius + 273; at T = 0 °K the pressure and volume of a gas are theoretically zero.)

b)   Ideal gas equation (universal gas law): $pV/T = constant$;
or $p_1 V_1/T_1 = p_2 V_2/T_2$.

For example, a mass of gas occupying 1 L at 127 °C is cooled to 27 °C and the pressure on the gas is halved. What is the new volume?
$p_1 V_1/T_1 = p_2 V_2/T_2$; we have $V_1 = 1$, $T_1 = 400$ K, $T_2 = 300$ K; inserting these values gives $p_1 \times 1/400 = 0.5p_1 \times V_2/300$ (T kelvin).
Finally: $0.5V_2 = 300 \div 400 = 0.75$, giving new volume $V_2 = 1.5$ L.

c)   Avagadro's law: $PV = nRT$ (R is the universal gas constant; n = no of moles = weight in grams ÷ molecular weight).

One mole of any gas occupies 22.4 litres at STP (where standard temperature and pressure is 0 °C and 1 atm). Note that one mole of any gas occupies 24 litres at RTP (room temperature and pressure).

d)   Dalton's law of partial pressures: $P_{total} = p_1 + p_2 + p_3$ etc.

For example, for air (nitrogen, oxygen, carbon dioxide): $P_{air} = pN_2 + pO_2 + pCO_2 + ...$
Composition of air: $N_2 = 78$ per cent; $O_2 = 21$ per cent; $CO_2 = 0.03$ per cent.
$P_{air} = 100$ kPa; so $pN_2 = 78$ kPa; $pO_2 = 21$ kPa; $pCO_2 = 0.03$ kPa.

e)   Gas transport (eg the lungs): at a constant temperature:

Henry's law: the solubility of a gas in contact with a liquid is proportional to its partial pressure.
Graham's law: the rate of diffusion of a gas is inversely proportional to the square root of its molecular mass.
Fick's first law: the rate of diffusion of a gas (across a membrane) is proportional to the surface area and the concentration gradient (difference in partial pressures across membrane), and inversely proportional to the distance (membrane thickness).

P15. Heat and energy

a)   Specific heat capacity (c) of a substance is the number of joules of heat energy (Q) required to raise the temperature of 1 g of the substance by 1 K. For water, $c = 4.2$ J g^{-1} K^{-1}.

The energy needed to raise m grams of a substance by ΔT degrees (K or °C; the increments of these two scales are the same, but their starting points are different) is given by: heat energy $Q = mc\Delta T$ joules.

For example, the heat energy required raise the temperature of 1 L of water from 25 °C to boiling point is given by: $Q = mc\Delta T = 1000 \times 4.2 \times (100 - 25)$ J $= 315$ kJ.

b)   Latent heat of vaporization (L) of a substance is the number of joules of heat energy (Q) required to change 1 g of the substance from liquid to vapour without change in temperature. For water, $L = 2260$ J g^{-1}.

The energy needed to convert m grams of a liquid to m grams of vapour at the same temperature is given by: heat of vaporization $= mL$ joules.

For example, the heat energy required to convert 1 L of water at 100 °C to steam at 100 °C is given by: $Q = mL = 1000 \times 2260$ J $= 2260$ kJ (ie seven times more energy than is required to reach boiling point).

c)   Latent heat of fusion (L) of a substance is the number of joules of heat energy (Q) required to change 1 g of the substance from solid to liquid without change in temperature. For water, $L = 334$ J g^{-1}. The energy needed to convert m grams of a solid to m grams of a liquid at the same temperature is given by: heat of fusion $= mL$ joules.

d)   Heat transfer: conduction (solids), convection (liquids; currents) and radiation (electromagnetic waves; black bodies emit and absorb the most wavelengths).

P16. Waves (light and sound)

a)   Two types: *transverse* (light and all electromagnetic waves; peaks, troughs) and *longitudinal* (eg sound; spring motion). Waves can be reflected at barriers (eg light at mirrors) and diffracted (bent) at corners and slits (eg sound waves).

b) $v = f\lambda$; v is the wave's speed (m s^{-1}), f its frequency (Hz; cycles s^{-1}), λ its wavelength (m). For light, $c = 3 \times 10^8$ m s$^{-1} = f\lambda$.

One wavelength is the distance between corresponding points on two successive waves (eg adjacent peaks), which is one cycle. Time for one cycle is the period (T) so we have $f = 1/T$ and $v = \lambda/T$. Amplitude (a) of wave $=$ *half the height between peak and trough*. Doppler: moving source; $v_s = 340$ m s^{-1} for sound (constant); wave appears shorter, frequency higher. Wave energy: $E = fh$ where E is in joules, f in hertz; h is Planck's constant (6.63×10^{-34} J Hz^{-1} or J s).

c)   Reflection: angle of incidence (i) $=$ angle of reflection (r); no change in velocity (same medium).

d)   Refraction: angle of incidence (i) $\neq$ angle of refraction (r); change in velocity (medium 1 to medium 2), wave bends (except when the wave strikes perpendicular to the boundary; then $i = r = 0°$). Refractive index (n): $n = \sin i/\sin r$ and $v_2/v_1 = \lambda_2/\lambda_1 = n_1/n_2 = \sin i/\sin r$; thus $n_1 \sin r = n_2 \sin i$.

Refractive index (n) for light in a medium is given by $n = c/v$ where c is the speed of light in a vacuum and v is the speed of light in the medium. A prism splits light because the constituent wavelengths travel at different speeds in glass but not in air. For example, air$_1$ to glass$_2$: light slows down, wavelength increases and light bends towards the normal.

Total internal reflection occurs when the critical angle of incidence is exceeded and all the light is reflected. The critical angle is given by: $i_{crit} = \sin^{-1} (n_1/n_2)$; (glass to air $n_2 > n_1$; $n_1 \sin r = n_2 \sin i$ with $r = 90°$, ie light travels parallel to interface).

e)   Lens formula: $1/u + 1/v = 1/f$; Lens magnification $M = v/u =$ ratio of object distance (v) to image distance (u); $f =$ focal length; $1/f = D$ (units $= m^{-1}$ or dioptres) $=$ lens power.

f)   Eye: short-sighted: distant light focused short of retina (lens too thick, ie too powerful; muscles not relaxed enough). Long-sighted: near light focused behind retina (lens too thin, ie not powerful enough; muscles too weak).

P17. Electrostatics, capacitance and electricity

a)   Coulomb's law: the electric forces of attraction (opposite charges) and repulsion (like charges) between two charged bodies (q_1 and q_2) are proportional to the inverse square of the distance of separation (r) and the product of the charges (distance $\times 2$ then force $\times 1/4$) $F = k\, q_1 q_2/r^2$ (k is the constant of proportionality). Positive charge flows outward; negative inward.

b)   Potential difference (volt): $1\, V = 1$ joule per coulomb.

c)   Capacitance (farad): capacitors are two parallel plates with equal and opposite charges ($\pm Q$), separated by insulating material (*dielectric* that supports an electrostatic field). Capacitance $=$ charge stored per volt: $C = Q/V$ or $Q = CV$. More charge is stored as the voltage increases, the plate separation decreases, the plate area increases and the dielectric constant of the insulator between plates increases. Energy (E joules) stored between the plates: $E = \frac{1}{2} CV^2$ (or the area under a charge voltage graph). Capacitors discharge exponentially; that is to say, a very high current flows at first, dropping away to zero (half-life $t_{1/2}$: 1/2 at t, $1/2 \times 1/2$ at $2t$), and across a resistor R, $t_{1/2}$ (s) $= \log_e (2) \times RC = 0.693 \times RC$ (logarithmic charge/discharge).

d) Current (I), voltage (V) and power (W):

amps = coulombs per second ($C\ s^{-1}$).
Thus 1 amp × 1 second = 1 coulomb of charge;
power = voltage × current = $J\ C^{-1} \times C\ s^{-1} = J\ s^{-1}$ = watt;
$W = VI$, and watt ($J\ s^{-1}$) × time (s) = energy (J) so:
energy = power × time (kW hours for household electricity).

e) Ohm's law (resistance), and power losses:

$V = IR$ (voltage current for a constant resistance R measured in ohms). Power loss (as heat energy) in a conductor of resistance R: $W = I^2R$ (substitute $V = IR$ in $W = VI$) so increase V to reduce I^2R losses (National Grid = 400 kV). Furthermore, R proportional to length of wire and inversely proportional to cross-sectional area ($diam^2$); thus longer, thinner wires offer more resistance.

P18. Kirchhoff's circuit laws, resistors and capacitors

a) Kirchhoff's current law: the current entering any point (node) in a circuit equals the current leaving it: $I_1 + I_2 + I_3 = I_4 + I_5 + I_6$.

b) Kirchhoff's voltage law (loop law): the sum of the changes in potential around any closed loop is zero; that is, the potential differences across any resistors must equal the potential difference across the battery (the latter is the electromotive force (EMF) of the battery ('battery voltage')). $V_{bat} = V_1 + V_2 + V_3$.
Thus $V_{bat} - V_1 - V_2 - V_3 = 0$. For example, work clockwise around a loop with the electricity flowing from positive to negative.

c) Resistors series (joined end to end, one end only): $R_{tot} = R_1 + R_2 + R_3$.

For a closed loop: the resistors have the same current passing through each of them: $V_{bat} = IR_1 + IR_2 + IR_3 = V_1 + V_2 + V_3$.

d) Resistors in parallel (joined to each other at both ends); reciprocal law:

$1/R_{tot} = 1/R_1 + 1/R_2 + 1/R_3$.
In a closed loop: each resistor has the same potential difference (ie equal to the battery voltage V_{bat}) and the current divides accordingly:
$I = I_1 + I_2 + I_3$ so $V_{bat}/R_{tot} = V_{bat}/R_1 + V_{bat}/R_2 + V_{bat}/R_3$.
NB: R_{tot} is always less than the smallest individual resistance.

e) Capacitors joined: the rules for combining capacitors are the opposite of those for combining resistors (use the reciprocal law for capacitors joined in series and the sum law for capacitors joined in parallel).

f)   Battery cells: for two (or more) cells wired in series (positive to negative), add the voltages together to find the resultant voltage. For two cells (of the same voltage) wired in parallel (positive to positive / negative to negative), the voltage remains unchanged. However, twice the amount of current can be supplied.

P19. Electromagnetism and electromagnetic induction

a)   Right-hand rule: a conductor (wire) carrying an electric current creates a magnetic field (flux) that radiates out in concentric circles. Grasp the wire with your right hand and point the thumb in the direction of the current; the magnetic field lines follow the rotation of your fingers around the wire.

b)   Magnetic force on a wire in a magnetic field is perpendicular to both the direction of current and the magnetic field; (open the fingers in a) above; palm of the hand faces the direction of force). Field strength (tesla T) is proportional to the current and inversely proportional to the distance from the wire. One T produces a force of 1 N per ampere per metre of wire.

Example i) motor: one side of the loops is attracted to the north poles of the magnets and the other sides to the south poles (rotates).
Example ii) solenoid: magnetic field runs parallel to the axis, giving north and south poles similar to a bar magnet.

c)   Electromagnetic induction (opposite of b)) in a conductor is an emf (and current) induced in a wire loop when the magnetic field changes (eg pushing a bar magnet into (or out of) a wire loop (or rotating the magnet), or changing the field strength in an electromagnet near the loop); current flows in a direction that opposes the change producing it. Examples include AC electrical generators.

d)   Transformers (electromagnetic induction): the primary AC voltage (V_1) is stepped down (or up) to the secondary AC voltage (V_2) by a factor equal to the ratio of the number of turns: secondary coil (N_2) to primary coil (N_1):
$V_2/V_1 = N_2 / N_1$ or $V_2 N_1 = V_1 N_2$.
Step-down transformer if N_2/N_1 less than 1. Step-up transformer if N_2/N_1 is greater than 1. The secondary power out equals the primary power in: $V_1 I_1 = V_2 I_2$; thus if the voltage is stepped down, the current is stepped up and vice versa; if the turns are stepped down, the current is stepped up and vice versa: $I_1 N_1 = I_2 N_2$.

P20. Radioactive decay

a)   Alpha, beta and gamma rays. *Alpha* particles are positively charged helium ions (helium atoms minus two electrons = nucleus = two protons and two neutrons); low penetration, stopped by paper; highly ionizing. *Beta* particles are high-energy electrons, stopped by thin aluminium; moderately ionizing. *Gamma* rays are high-energy photons (electromagnetic radiation; $E = f\,h$); high penetration, stopped by several centimetres of dense metal (eg lead); weakly ionizing.

For example, alpha decay: (lose charge +2, mass 4): $^{238}_{92}U$ to $^{234}_{90}Th + {}^{4}_{2}He$;
beta decay: (lose charge −1, mass 0): $^{90}_{38}Sr$ to $^{90}_{39}Y + {}^{0}_{-1}e$;
(mass change = 0; neutron decays to a proton, emits an electron);
gamma decay (charge and mass unchanged): $^{12}_{6}C$ to $^{12}_{7}N + \gamma ray$.

b)   Half-life ($T_{1/2}$): radioactive isotopes (radioisotopes) decay spontaneously to produce alpha or beta particles. The number of disintegrations is proportional to the number of active atoms left (exponential decay). For example, radio-active iodine (iodine-131) can be used to treat thyroid cancer. The half-life is eight days. The number of active atoms continues to halve for every half-life elapsed from the time of preparation (from time/day 0).

For example, what percentage of a sample of radioactive iodine-131 (half-life = 8 days) remains undecayed (ie active) after eight weeks?
8 weeks = 56 days; 56 days ÷ 8 days per half-life = 7 half-lives; the fraction remaining is: $1/2 \times 1/2 \times 1/2 \times 1/2 \times 1/2 \times 1/2 \times 1/2$ (or $(1/2)^7$) = 1/128 = 0.78 per cent (to 2 sf).

c)   One becquerel (Bq) = 1 atom disintegrating per second (1 count per second).

d)   One electron volt (eV) is the kinetic energy acquired by an electron losing one volt of potential.

Physics review questions

Q1   (P4c) A man falls from a ladder and lands on the ground exactly 0.5 seconds later. How far did he fall? Gravity is 10 m s^{-2}.

(hint: $ut + \frac{1}{2}at^2$)

Answer [＿＿＿＿＿]

Q2   (P6e) A stone is thrown horizontally from a vertical cliff at a speed of 20 metres per second. The cliff is 30 metres above sea level and the stone hits the sea after 2.5 seconds. How far from the base of the cliff is the stone when it hits the sea? $g = 10$ m s^{-2}?

(hint: treat horizontal and vertical motion separately)

Answer [＿＿＿＿＿]

Q3   (P7a,b,e,f) A rightward force is applied to a 10-kg object to move it across a rough surface at constant velocity. The coefficient of friction between the object and the surface is 0.2.

Use the diagram to determine the following forces: ($g = 10$ m s^{-2})

(hint: Newton's three laws: acceleration?)

A. gravitational force
B. normal force
C. friction force
D. applied force

Answer [＿＿＿＿＿]

Q4   (P7c,g) A parachutist of mass 80 kg reaches a terminal velocity of 50 m s^{-1}, at which point he throws a ball vertically downwards at a velocity of 20 m s^{-1} relative to him. What is the acceleration of the ball vertically downwards relative to the parachutist immediately after it has been thrown? (1 kg = 10 N.)

A. 0 m s^{-2}
B. 70 m s^{-1}
C. 30 m s^{-1}
D. 10 m s^{-2}

(hint: units)

Answer _____

Q5   (P8b) A hydraulic ramp can lift a vehicle weighing 6 tonnes to a height of 2 metres in 50 seconds. What is the power of the ramp in kilowatts? (1 kg = 10 N.)

(hint: rate of work)

Answer _____

Q6   (P8c) At a hydroelectric pumped storage scheme, the reservoir is 500 metres above the turbine house. What is the velocity of the water when it arrives at the turbines? Neglect energy losses on the descent and take *g* to be 10 m s^{-2}.

(hint: conservation of energy)

Answer _____

Q7   (P8a, 17c) An electric scooter has a mass of 100 kg (including its user). The force required to overcome its rolling resistance is 10 per cent of its weight. It is driven by a 24-volt electric motor that takes its power from batteries that hold 2×10^5 coulombs of charge. What is the range of the scooter in kilometres? (1 kg = 10 N.)

(hint: work done by scooter = work done by batteries)

Answer _____

Q8   (P16b) The frequency of middle C on the piano is 260 Hz. If sound waves travel at a speed of 338 m s^{-1}, what is the wavelength of middle C in centimetres?

A. 125 cm
B. 130 cm
C. 132 cm
D. 131 cm
E. 128 cm

(hint: units; cycles per sec)

Answer ⬚

Q9   (P7e, 10a,b) A 12-gauge shotgun weighing 6 kg fires 30 g of lead shot at 400 m s^{-1}. What is the speed of recoil of the gun?

(hint: momentum)

Answer ⬚

Q10   (P17d) What is the power of an electric kettle if the heating element has a resistance of 23 ohm? Take mains voltage to be 230 volts.

A. 2.2 kW
B. 2.3 kW
C. 2.5 kW
D. 3 kW
E. 1.5 kW

(hint: Ohm's law)

Answer ⬚

Q11   (P17d) How much energy does a 3-kilowatt electric kettle consume when it is connected to a 240-volt supply for three minutes?

(hint: ignore voltage)

Answer ⬚

Q12 (P5) Which pair of the graphs below could show the motion of the same object?

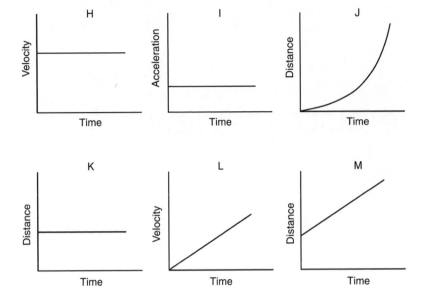

A. L and M
B. H and K
C. L and M
D. J and L
E. J and M

Answer _____

Chemistry review

C1.   Atoms, electron configuration and valency
C2.   Periodic table
C3.   Bonding: electrovalent (ionic), covalent and metallic
C4.   The mole and balancing chemical equations (reactions)
C5.   Types of chemical reaction
C6.   Concentration and pH; reaction rates
C7.   Exothermic and endothermic reactions; Le Chatelier's principle
C8.   Solids, liquids, gases; changes of state; thermochemistry
C9.   Electrochemistry, reactivity series and electrolysis
C10.   Carbon (organic) chemistry; fractional distillation
        Chemistry review questions

C1. Atoms, electron configuration and valency

a) Atomic number: the number of protons in the atom

Neutral atoms: number of protons (+) = number of electrons (−).

b) Atomic mass

Number of protons + number of neutrons; usually more than twice atomic number (C, N, O, S, Si, Mg, Ca are exactly ×2).
The atomic mass is written above the atomic number, eg $^{12}_{6}C$.

c) Electron config: quantum number (n) of electron shells

$n = 1$ (2 electrons max in 1 subshell type) $1s^2$.
$n = 2$ (8 electrons max in 2 subshell types) $2s^2\,2p^6$.
$n = 3$ (18 electrons max in 3 subshell types) $3s^2\,3p^6\,3d^{10}$.
$n = 4$ (32 electrons max in 4 subshell types) $4s^2\,4p^6\,4d^{10}\,4f^{14}$.

s-p-d-f; fill the lowest energy levels first s2, p6, d10, f14:
　　　for example, iron: atomic number 26: $1s^2\,2s^2\,2p^6\,3s^2\,3p^6\,4s^2\,3d^6$;
　　　silver: atomic number 47: $1s^2\,2s^2\,2p^6\,3s^2\,3p^6\,4s^2\,3d^{10}\,4p^6\,5s^2\,4d^9$.

d) Valency

The number of valence (outer) shell electrons an atom must lose or gain to achieve a valence octet (8 = noble gas structure). Atoms combine to achieve full shells.
　　For example, sodium: atomic number 11: $2 + 8 + 1$ ($1s^2\,2s^2\,2p^6\,3s^1$);
　　chlorine: atomic number 17: $2 + 8 + 7$ ($1s^2\,2s^2\,2p^6\,3s^2\,3p^5$).

$Na^+ = 2 + 8$; $Cl^- = 2 + 8 + 8$. For Na: $1s^2\,2s^2\,2p^6\,3s^1 =$ ground state;
$1s^2\,2s^2\,2p^6 =$ ionized state; $1s^2\,2s^1\,2p^6\,3s^2 =$ (photon) excited state.

e) Periodic table

Groups = vertical columns; periods = rows; periods correspond with principal quantum number; same group elements have the same valency/similar properties. Reactivity:

Group 1: alkali metals: Li < Na < K < Rb < Cs; (form cations^{+1}).
Group 2: alkaline earth metals: Be < Mg < Ca < Sr < Ba (form cations^{+2}).
Group 13: B, Al (form cations^{+3}).
Group 14: C, Si.
Group 15: N, P (form anions^{-3}).
Group 16: O, S (form anions^{-2}).
Group 17: halogens: F > Cl > Br > I; (form anions^{-1}).
Group 18: (or 0) noble gases: He, Ne, Ar (inert, octet; eg 2,8,8).

Charges balance in compounds, eg calcium chloride $Ca^{2+}(Cl^-)_2$.

C2. Periodic table

C2 Periodic Table (short form; 4 periods: 1 to 4 electron shells; 18 groups)

smaller atoms, more electronegative (left to right and bottom to top) ⟶

1																	$^{1}_{1}H$						$^{4}_{2}He$

p-block

| 2 | $^{7}_{3}Li$ | $^{9}_{4}Be$ | | | | | | | | | | $^{11}_{5}B$ | $^{12}_{6}C$ | $^{14}_{7}N$ | $^{16}_{8}O$ | $^{19}_{9}F$ | $^{20}_{10}Ne$ |

| 3 | $^{23}_{11}Na$ | $^{24}_{12}Mg$ | | | d-block | | | | | | | $^{27}_{13}Al$ | $^{28}_{14}Si$ | $^{31}_{15}P$ | $^{32}_{16}S$ | $^{35.5}_{17}Cl$ | $^{40}_{18}Ar$ |

| 4 | $^{39}_{19}K$ | $^{40}_{20}Ca$ | $^{45}_{21}Sc$ | $^{48}_{22}Ti$ | $^{51}_{23}V$ | $^{52}_{24}Cr$ | $^{55}_{25}Mn$ | $^{56}_{26}Fe$ | $^{59}_{27}Co$ | $^{59}_{28}Ni$ | $^{64}_{29}Cu$ | $^{65}_{30}Zn$ | $^{70}_{31}Ga$ | $^{73}_{32}Ge$ | $^{75}_{33}As$ | $^{79}_{34}Se$ | $^{80}_{35}Br$ | $^{84}_{36}Kr$ |

s-block   non-metals ⟶

s-block (alkali metals; soft metals, very reactive, not found in the free state, reducing agents (donate electrons), dissolve in water to give alkaline solutions; alkaline earth metals; light metals, water insoluble)

p-block (eg halogens; metal halides are crystalline, water soluble, oxidizing agents eg F (accept electrons) (eg noble gases; colourless and unreactive with stable electronic configurations (octet))

d-block (transition metals; high strength, high melting points, form coloured compounds)

Chlorine-35.5 is the weighted average of two **isotopes** Cl-35 (18 neutrons) and Cl-37 (20 neutrons)

Definitions: Cl is an **element** made up of **atoms**; Cl_2 is a **molecule** (a discrete unit of atoms bonded); an unreacted **mixture** of H_2 and Cl_2 exposed to sunlight react to form a **compound** (HCl); Cl^{-1} is an **ion**

C3. Bonding: electrovalent (ionic), covalent and metallic

a) Electrovalent (ionic)

Atoms exchange electrons to give ions that form strong electrostatic bonds (positive cations, negative anions). Bond strength increases with increasing charge and smaller ions (fluoride smallest anion, lithium smallest cation). Properties: inorganic salts with giant lattice structures (ionic crystals); solid at room temperature with high melting and boiling points (strong bonds); conduct electricity when molten or dissolved in water (ionic solution); iodides most soluble (dissociate) in water, fluorides least soluble. Insoluble in organic solvents. Examples: groups 1, 2 metal halides ($Na^{+}Cl^{-}$, $Ca^{2+}F_2^{-}$).

b) Covalent

Atoms share one or more electron pairs to achieve full shells (eight outer electrons) as per the following diatomic and triatomic *molecules*: H_2, Cl_2, F_2, N_2, O_2, CO; H_2O, H_2S, CO_2, NO_2.

The number of shared electron pairs is the molecular covalency.

Carbon has four outer electrons ($2s^2\ 2p^2$) and attains a valency of four ($2s^2\ 2p^6$) by sharing with another four pairs; for example CH_4 = four single covalent bonds, CO_2 = two double covalent bonds. Properties: opposite of ionic; low melting/boiling points (eg gas); non-conducting; 'like dissolves like' so some are soluble in organic (C-based) solvents such as ethanol, but insoluble in water.

c) Metallic

Atoms are packed together tightly (like snooker balls in a triangle), surrounded by a sea of electrons (de-localized).

Properties: most have high melting points (strong bonds); good electrical and thermal conductivity (highly mobile outer electrons); high strength, especially when alloyed with other metals (eg brass = 60 per cent copper and 40 per cent tin).

d) Electronegativity

This is the ability of atoms to attract electrons; concept links ionic and covalent bonding. A large difference (>2) favours ionic bonds (eg Cl high, Na low) whereas similar electronegativities favour covalent bonds (eg C, H); intermediate (eg Cl and H) form polar compounds that display both types of bonding (HCl is a covalent gas that forms aqueous ions).

C4. The mole and balancing chemical equations (reactions)

a) Mole

By *definition* one mole of any substance contains 6.022×10^{23} particles of the substance (Avogadro's number); for example, 'one mole of peanuts contains 6.022×10^{23} peanuts'. More usefully, 6.022×10^{23} atoms, ions or molecules is one mole of each. For an element, an amount in grams equal to the atomic mass contains one mole of atoms. For a molecule such as H_2O, one mole of H_2O contains two moles of H and one mole of O. The molecular mass of H_2O is $2 + 16 = 18$ so 18 grams of H_2O = 1 mole H_2O ($2 \times 6.022 \times 10^{23}$ atoms of H and $1 \times 6.022 \times 10^{23}$ atoms of O).

More generally: mass ÷ molecular mass = number of moles;

for example, 54 grams of water is $54 \div 18 = 3$ moles of water.

b) Balancing chemical equations

Atoms are neither created nor destroyed, so where we have same number of atoms on each side of the equation.

For example, $H_2 + O_2 = H_2O$ (unbalanced; two hydrogens + two oxygens on the left but two hydrogens + one oxygen on the right). We have one too many oxygen atoms on the left so to balance:

$H_2 + \frac{1}{2} O_2 = H_2O$ and normally written as $2H_2 + O_2 \rightarrow 2H_2O$.

For more complicated equations:

i)   Balance the atoms in the more complex molecules first. Try the molecule on the far left of the equation (balance the atoms in this molecule with the same atoms on the right of the equation).

ii) Balance the simpler molecules second, leaving the diatomic molecules (1 atom type) until the last (eg hydrogen, oxygen).

For example, in the combustion of propane with oxygen the following reaction takes place:

$C_3H_8 + O_2 \rightarrow CO_2 + H_2O$ (skeleton equation).

i)   Starting with propane on the left; it has 3 carbon atoms to be balanced:

$C_3H_8 + O_2 \rightarrow 3CO_2 + H_2O$; now balance the 8 H atoms:

$C_3H_8 + O_2 \rightarrow 3CO_2 + 4H_2O$.

ii) Finally, balance the O atoms: $C_3H_8 + 5O_2 \rightarrow 3CO_2 + 4H_2O$
(3 carbon, 8 hydrogen and 10 oxygen atoms on each side).

C5. Types of chemical reaction

a) Neutralization

- acid (H^+) + base (OH^-) → metal salt + water.

  (base = metal oxide/hydroxide and if soluble → alkali eg NaOH.)

- acid + carbonate/hydrogen carbonate → metal salt + water + CO_2.

- acid + ammonia → ammonium salt + water.

- acid + metal → metal salt + hydrogen.

b) Oxidation-reduction (redox)

For every oxidation there is a corresponding reduction.

- Oxidation = add oxygen/remove hydrogen/loss of electrons.

- Reduction = remove oxygen/add hydrogen/gain of electrons.

('OILRIG' – oxidation is loss; reduction is gain).

For a redox reaction: valency = oxidation number (+ or –) and the charges balance on either side of the equation.

- $Fe + CuSO_4 \rightarrow FeSO_4 + Cu$; split into half-reactions:

- $Fe \rightarrow Fe^{2+} + 2e^-$ (oxidation; Fe oxidation number 0 to +2);

- $Cu^{2+} + 2e^- \rightarrow Cu$ (reduction; Cu oxidation number +2 to 0);

- Fe (reducing agent) oxidized; Cu^{2+} (oxidizing agent) reduced.

c) Displacement reaction

Single: $Fe + CuSO_4 \rightarrow FeSO_4 + Cu$ (replacement; also a redox);
Double: $FeS + 2HCl \rightarrow FeCl_2 + H_2S$ (2 new compounds formed).

d) Combustion reaction

The oxidation of each element in the compound; for example, a hydrocarbon fuel burning in O_2.

e) Composition, decomposition and dissociation

Composition (synthesis) $A + B \rightarrow AB$; decomposition: $AB \rightarrow A + B$; dissociation: $AB \rightarrow A^+ + B^-$ (eg NaCl in water).

Composition one way, decomposition the other: $2H + O_2 = H_2O$.

f) Substitution

Swap an atom, ion or group in a molecule; for example, swap a hydrogen linked to a carbon: $CH_4 + Cl_2 \rightarrow CH_3Cl + HCl$.

g) Hydrolysis/condensation

Hydrolysis = add water molecule; condensation = remove water molecule.

C6. Concentration and pH; reaction rates

a) Concentration: moles per dm³ (litre)

1 mole of solute in 1 litre of solution = 1.0 molar (M) solution. Normality (N) is used with acids (or alkalis) to reflect the number of protons (or hydroxide ions) per litre.
    For example 1.0 M H_2SO_4 = 2.0 N H_2SO_4; 1.0 M = 1.0 N for HCl, NaOH.

Medicine uses millimoles per litre (mmol/L); for example blood: glucose 4 to 6 mmol/L, Na 135–145 mmol/L, K 3.5–5 mmol/L, cholesterol 5 mmol/L. (NB 'Normal saline' for infusions is 0.9 per cent weight/volume (w/v) NaCl (ie 0.9 g NaCl per 100 ml of water; not Normality)).

b) pH scale ('potential of hydrogen')

pH = $-\log_{10}$ moles H^+/L.
pH ranges from pH 0 (strong acid) to pH 14 (strong alkali).

● pH H_2O = 7 (neutral). Log scale (× 10, × 100, × 1000 H^+ etc).

● 0.1 M HCl, pH = $-\log_{10}$ 0.1 = 1; 0.01 M HCl, pH = $-\log_{10}$ 0.01 = 20.

● 001 M HCl, pH = $-\log_{10}$ 0.001 = 3.0; pH gastric HCl approx 1 to 2.

● H_2O = H^+ + OH^-; $[H^+]$ = 10^{-7} pH = $-\log_{10}10^{-7}$ = 7 (neutral).

$[H^+]$ = $[OH^-]$ = 10^{-7}; equilibrium constant K_w = product of the concentrations, that is to say K_w = $[H^+][OH^-]$ = 10^{-14} so if add acid (H^+) to water pH goes down and pOH (hydroxide ions) goes up; eg if pH = 5, pOH = 9.

c) Reaction rates

For A + B = product; rate = k $[A]^x$ $[B]^y$.

i) Rate: product of concentrations A, B and the *order* of the reaction:
    zero-order reaction ($x + y = 0$): rate = k (k is the rate constant);
    first-order reaction ($x + y = 1$): rate = $k[A]$ or k $[B]$;
    second-order reaction ($x + y = 2$): rate = $k[A]^2$, k $[B]^2$ or $k[A][B]$.

ii) Rate increases with increasing temperature (approx $\times 2$ for every 10 °C rise in temperature). Molecules have more kinetic energy; a greater proportion overcome the activation energy (ie the height of the peak on a potential-energy/reaction graph).

iii) Rate increases in the presence of a catalyst (eg enzyme) that lowers the activation energy for the reaction. Faster equilibrium but position unchanged. Catalysts not consumed.

iv) Rate increases with greater surface area (eg powder).

C7. Exothermic and endothermic reactions; Le Chatelier's principle

a) Exothermic reactions

Heat energy is released. Enthalpy of reaction is negative; $\Delta H < 0$ (gives off heat/lost to surroundings). Examples: combustion and bond making (gets hotter):

$$CH_{4(g)} + 2O_{2(g)} \rightarrow CO_{2(g)} + 2H_2O_{(g)} \qquad \Delta H = -890 \text{ kJ mol}^{-1};$$
$$N_{2(g)} + 3H_{2(g)} \rightarrow 2NH_{3(g)} \qquad \Delta H = -90 \text{ kJ mol}^{-1}.$$

b) Endothermic reactions

Heat energy is absorbed. Enthalpy of reaction is positive; $\Delta H > 0$ (heat added from surroundings). Examples: liquid to gas and bond breaking (cools down):

$$H_2O_{(l)} \rightarrow H_2O_{(g)} \qquad \Delta H = +43 \text{ kJ mol}^{-1}.$$
$$2NH_{3(g)} \rightarrow N_{2(g)} + 3H_{2(g)} \qquad \Delta H = +90 \text{ kJ mol}^{-1}.$$

Reversible reaction: $N_{2(g)} + 3H_{2(g)} = 2NH_{3(g)}$ (a dynamic equilibrium): that is, exothermic to the right and endothermic to the left.

c) Le Chatelier's principle

For a system in equilibrium, when a change is made to the conditions the equilibrium will shift so as to oppose the change.

● Temperature: raise it and the reaction shifts to absorb heat; lower it and the reaction shifts to produce more heat.

Endothermic reaction: raise the temperature, equilibrium moves to the left to absorb excess heat (more $N_{2(g)} + 3H_{2(g)}$).

Exothermic reactions: lower the temperature and the equilibrium moves to the right to produce more heat (more NH_3).

- Pressure: increase it and the reaction shifts to lower it (by reducing the number of molecules/volume) and vice versa.

   For example $N_{2(g)} + 3H_{2(g)} = 2NH_{3(g)}$ (1 mole + 3 moles = 2 moles).
   Increase the pressure to produce more NH_3.

- Concentration: increase the concentration of a molecule and the reaction shifts to decrease it and vice versa. Add N_2, H_2, or remove NH_3 and the equilibrium shifts to the right (more NH_3). NB: do not confuse equilibrium ('how far') and reaction rates ('how fast'); in NH_3 production, a low temperature would favour a greater proportion (yield) but the reaction is too slow; so 500 °C, 300 atmospheres, add a catalyst to increase the rate (no effect on equilibrium) and remove the NH_3 as it is produced.

C8. Solids, liquids, gases; changes of state; thermochemistry

a) Gases, liquids, solids

i) **Gases:** very low density; no shape, weak bonds; particles diffuse to fill any volume; easy to compress. Pressure of a gas is a linear function of temperature. *PV* is constant at constant temperature (see Physics P14).

ii) **Liquids:** much more dense than gases and usually less dense than when in the solid state (water/ice is the notable exception). Constant volume (incompressible for most practical purposes, eg hydraulic rams); take on the shape of the container; particles are bonded locally. Expand much less than gases when heated.

iii) **Solids:** usually the most dense state and incompressible, though depends on the structure. Strong bonds between particles, so take on a rigid form. Expand less than liquids on heating. All metals, mercury excepted, are solids at room temperature.

b) Changes of state (gas, liquid and solid)

i) **Solid to liquid, liquid to solid:** solid to liquid = melting point (heat energy absorbed) and liquid to solid = freezing point (reverse of melting at the same temperature, heat released); liquid to gas = vaporization (heat absorbed) and gas to liquid = condensation (heat released); also solid to gas = sublimation; gas to solid = deposition.

Examples: ice at 0 °C melts to water at 0 °C with heat in, and water at 0 °C freezes to (wet) ice at 0 °C with heat out; water boils at 100 °C and vaporizes to steam at 100 °C with heat in, and steam at 100 °C condenses to water at 100 °C with heat out; dry ice (solid carbon dioxide) sublimes to carbon dioxide gas. NB: evaporation is vaporization at the surface of the liquid, whereas boiling is vaporization from within the body of the liquid as well.

ii) **Temperature versus pressure graph:** solid to liquid to gas with increasing temperature and gas to liquid to solid with increasing pressure (which increases the boiling point). Triple point: all three states in equilibrium; critical temperature: above this a gas cannot be condensed to liquid by increased pressure.

iii) **Impurities:** impurities such as grit or salt lower the freezing point (snow melts in the presence of rock salt) and increase the boiling point.

C9. Electrochemistry, reactivity series and electrolysis

a) Electrochemistry

Chemical reactions can give rise to electricity (batteries) and vice versa (electrolysis of electrolytes).

i)   Conductors: metals, and carbon in the form of graphite.

ii) Insulators: non-metals (glass/ceramics, polymers, rubber).

iii) Semi-conductors: (between i, ii) silicon 'chips' (metalloids).

iv) Electrolytes: conduct electricity when molten or dissolved in water (eg salts, acids, alkalis).

v)   Electrodes: positive (anode) and negative (cathode) terminals.

b) Electrolysis

When an electrical current is passed through an electrolyte, cations migrate to the cathode, where electrons are added (reduction), and anions migrate to the anode, where electrons are removed/lost (oxidation); an example is the electrolytic extraction of Al: molten cryolite (sodium aluminium fluoride at 1000 °C, 5 volt, 30 kA):

- at the cathode (negative): $Al^{3+} + 3e^- = Al$ (charges balance);

- at the anode (positive): $2O^{2-} = O_2 + 4e^-$ (charges balance).

Faraday's law of electrolysis states that the amount of aluminium deposited at the cathode, or oxygen liberated at the anode, is directly proportional to the amount of current passed.

1 faraday (F) = 1 mole of electrons = 96 500 coulombs.

So 3 moles of electrons (3 faradays) will deposit 1 mole of aluminium (27 g) from 1 mole of Al^{3+} cations and 0.75 moles of oxygen (12g) from 2 moles of O^{2-} anions. 1 coulomb of charge = 1 amp for 1 second so 96 500 ampere seconds will deposit one-third of a mole of aluminium (9 g).

c) Reactivity series

i)   K, Na, Ca, Mg, Al, C, Zn, Fe, Sn, Pb, H, Cu, Ag, Au, Pt. More electropositive (reactive) metals displace less electropositive (more noble) metals from solution (eg iron displaces copper from copper sulphate).

ii)   Electrolysis of salts in water: metals above/before H (more reactive) are not formed at the cathode; instead H_2 is discharged. At the anode O_2 is discharged, except for halides salts (when halogen is discharged instead). Summary: O_2 at anode unless halide salt (halogen discharged); H_2 at cathode, unless Cu^{2+} (then Cu deposited).

iii)   Electrolysis of acids: dilute solutions give H_2 and O_2 (2:1 volume ratio); concentrated hydrochloric acid gives H_2 and Cl_2 (1:1 volume ratio).

C10. Carbon (organic) chemistry; fractional distillation

a) Allotropes of carbon

Carbon has three main allotropes: graphite, carbon and fullerenes (buckyball); in other words, the same element occurs in a different physical form with a different molecular structure.

i)   Graphite: an electrically conducting soft powder; giant non-crystalline sheets that slide over each other (three strong covalent bonds in 2-d hexagonal planes and one weak bond between planes).

ii) Diamond: very hard; giant structure with four strong covalent bonds.

iii) Fullerenes: hollow spherical clusters of carbon atoms such as C_{60}.

b) Alkanes, alkenes, alkynes

i) Alkanes (C_nH_{2n+2}): carbon–carbon single bonds (eg methane CH_4, propane C_3H_8); saturated hydrocarbons (C, H only); combust completely in air to produce water and carbon dioxide, or carbon monoxide if combustion incomplete (lack of oxygen).

ii) Alkenes (C_nH_{2n}): carbon–carbon double bonds (eg ethane, C_2H_4).

iii) Alkynes (C_nH_{2n-2}): carbon–carbon triple bonds (eg propyne, C_3H_4).

c) Fractional distillation

Fractional distillation (ie evaporation and condensation) separates a mixture (compounds that are not combined chemically) into its constituents according to their boiling points. In the fractional distillation of crude oil, the alkanes with shorter carbon chains (<10 carbons) are lighter, boil off first and are highly flammable (eg propane); the larger molecules (carbon chains > 20) are less volatile, highly viscous (flow less easily) and are more difficult to ignite (eg heavy fuel oil, bitumen).

i) Cracking (with steam) breaks less useful, longer hydrocarbon chains into more useful shorter chains; for example, heavy fuel oil to petrol.

ii) Polymerization of alkenes (unsaturated hydrocarbons) builds short chains to long chains; for example, ethene to polyethene (polyethylene).

iii) Reforming changes straight chain hydrocarbons into aromatic hydrocarbons; for example, hexane to benzene (same number of carbons).

iv) Isomers have the same formula but a different arrangement of atoms; for example, 2-methyl-propane is an isomer of butane; both are C_4H_{10}. Isomers may have different physical/chemical properties.

Chemistry review questions

Q1   (C1, 2) Silicon is found in group 14 of the periodic table.

Silicon-30 is an isotope of silicon. Which of the following statements is true for silicon-30?

A. 14 protons, 14 neutrons and 14 electrons.
B. 14 protons, 16 neutrons and 14 electrons.
C. 16 protons, 14 neutrons and 16 electrons.
D. 30 neutrons plus protons and 16 electrons.

Answer [   ]

Q2   (C4a) An organic compound is combusted and found to contain 36 per cent carbon, 6 per cent hydrogen and 48 per cent oxygen by mass. Which of the following is the correct chemical formula of the compound?

A. $C_2H_4O_2$
B. $C_4H_{10}O$
C. $C_3H_6O_3$
D. $C_6H_{12}O_4$
E. $C_2H_2O_2$

(hint: take 100 g)

Answer [   ]

Q3   (C4a) How many dm³ (litres) of carbon dioxide are produced if 200 ml of 1.0 molar (1 M) hydrochloric acid is added to 0.5 moles of calcium carbonate? (1 mole of any gas occupies 24 dm³ at RTP.)

$$CaCO_3 + 2HCl = CaCl_2 + H_2O + CO_2.$$

A. 24

B. 12

C. 2.4

D. 1.2

(hint: 1.0 M = 1 mole per litre)

Answer

Q4   (C4b) The body burns glucose with oxygen to release energy. The end products are carbon dioxide and water. What values of *a*, *b* and *c* are needed to balance the equation?

$$C_6H_{12}O_6 + aO_2 = bCO_2 + cH_2O.$$

(hint: *b* first)

a = ...

b = ...

c = ...

Q5   (C5ii) In which of the following compounds does carbon have the lowest oxidation number?

A. CF_4

B. CH_4

C. C_2H_6

D. CF_3

E. C

(hint: 0, –, +)

Answer

Q6   (C4a) A dehydrated patient is prescribed 1.0 L Normal saline (9 g/L NaCl), given by subcutaneous infusion over eight hours. Which of the following calculations describes the number of millimoles of sodium infused? The AMU of sodium (atomic mass unit) is 23 and the AMU of chlorine is 35.5.

A. $9 \div (23 \div 58.5) \times 1000 = 6.7$ mmol
B. $9 \div 23 \times 1000 = 391.3$ mmol
C. $9 \div (23 \div 35.5) \times 1000 = 11.0$ mmol
D. $9 \div (23 + 35.5) \times 1000 = 153.8$ mmol

(hint: NaCl molecular mass)

Answer [   ]

Q7   (C5ii) In photographic fixing, sodium thiosulphate removes unexposed silver bromide according to the following equation:

$$AgBr + 2[Na_2(S_2O_3)^{2-}] \rightarrow Na_3[Ag(S_2O_3)_2]^{3-} + NaBr$$

Which of the following statements describes correctly the behaviour of the silver in the equation?

A. Ag is oxidized from +1 to +3 and acts as a reducing agent.
B. Ag is oxidized from +1 to +3 and acts as an oxidizing agent.
C. Ag is reduced from +1 to 0 and acts as an oxidizing agent.
D. Ag is oxidized from −1 to 0 and acts as a reducing agent.

(hint: Na cations)

Answer [   ]

Q8   (C5c, C6) Sulphur dioxide reacts with oxygen to produce sulphur trioxide according to the following equilibrium:

$$2SO_{2(g)} + O_{2(g)} = 2SO_{3(g)} \qquad \Delta H = -390 \text{ kJ}.$$

Which one of the following changes moves the equilibrium most in favour of sulphur trioxide?

A. Increase temperature and increase pressure.
B. Increase temperature and increase reactant concentrations.
C. Increase temperature and add a catalyst.
D. Decrease temperature and add a catalyst.
E. Decrease temperature and increase pressure.

(hint: not rate)

Answer [   ]

Q9 (C6a,b) Which of the following aqueous solutions will have a pH of approximately 10?

A. 1 M sodium chloride.
B. 0.01 M hydrochloric acid.
C. 0.001 M sulphuric acid.
D. 0.001 M sodium hydroxide.
E. 0.0001 M potassium hydroxide.

(hint: $[H^+][OH^-] = 10^{-14}$)

Answer _____

Q10 (C9) The apparatus below shows the electrolysis of copper sulphate solution using carbon (inert) electrodes. Choose the correct term, substance or equation (labelled A to E) from the list below to match each label on the diagram (i to iv).

A = oxidation;   B = reduction;   C = $Cu^{2+} + 2e^- = Cu$;   D = O_2;   E = Cl_2.

i) = ...
ii) = ...
iii) = ...
iv) = ...

Q11 (C9, P14a, P15) The graph shows the time–temperature curve of pure ice when heated.

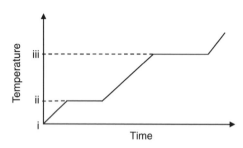

Which of the following statements are true and which are false?

A. There are three phases with two phase changes in between.
B. The temperature at i is 273 K.
C. Water is boiling between temperatures ii and iii.
D. The temperature at iii is 373 K.
E. The water temperature rises by 100 K between ii and iii.

Q12 (C10c) Choose the chemical formula (labelled A to I) from the list below to match each numbered space (i to v) in the following text. Some formulae are not used.

$A = C_2H_6$; $B = C_8H_{18}$; $C = C_{10}H_{22}$; $D = CH_3OH$; $E = C_2H_4Br_2$; $F = HBr$;
$G = C_2H_4$; $H = C_2H_5Br$; $I = Br_2$.

In cracking, [...i...] is broken down into [...ii...] and ethene [...iii...]. Ethene is unsaturated and it will react with [...iv...] to produce the colourless liquid 1,2-dibromoethane [...v...].

i)   = ...

ii) = ...

iii) = ...

iv) = ...

v)   = ...

ew

trual cycle hormones

cid), genes and cell division

s

B1. Digestive system

a) Passage of food

Mouth, tongue, pharynx (throat), oesophagus (food pipe), stomach, small intestine (duodenum, ileum) and large intestine (colon, rectum).

b) Nutrients and catalytic enzymes

i)   Carbohydrates: (polysaccharides) digested with salivary amylase
     (to disaccharides (eg maltose) and monosaccharides (eg glucose)).

ii) Proteins: digested with pepsin, trypsin and chymotrypsin in the stomach
     (to polypeptides and amino acids).

iii) Fats: digested with bile salts (emulsify/solubulize) and pancreatic amylase,
     trypsin and lipase (to fatty acids and glycerol). Most absorption of nutrients
     takes place in the small intestine via the blood capillaries of villi
     (large surface area).

Enzymes (protein molecules) are food specific and have an optimum pH (pH 2 in
stomach; pH 7 in the mouth and small intestine; eg salivary amylase stops working
in the stomach) and work best at body temperature (37 °C; denature above 45 °C). The
digestive tract is lubricated with mucus, which protects it from the digestive enzymes.
Water is absorbed by the large intestine and indigestible material is eliminated.

B2. Respiratory system

a) Air pathway

Nose, nasal cavity, pharynx (throat) larynx (voice box), trachea (windpipe), two bronchi
(one bronchus enters each lung), bronchioles and alveoli.

b) Respiration

i)   Breathing (pulmonary ventilation): the physical process of inspiration/expiration:
     on *inspiration* the diaphragm and intercostal muscles *contract*, the diaphragm
     moves down, the thoracic volume increases, the pressure decreases and air is
     drawn into the lungs. On *expiration* the muscles *relax*, the diaphragm moves
     upwards, the thoracic volume decreases, the thoracic pressure increases and
     the lungs deflate.

ii) External respiration: the exchange of oxygen and carbon dioxide in the lungs
     between the alveoli and the pulmonary capillaries. *Diffusion* of gases in the
     alveoli is aided by a large surface area, thin walls, moist lining and good blood
     supply. Oxygen is carried to respiring cells by red blood cells (RBCs);
     haemoglobin (Hb) in RBCs binds four molecules of oxygen as oxyhaemoglobin
     (HbO_8); carbon dioxide from respiring cells is carried away as hydrogen
     carbonate ions.

iii)   Internal respiration: cellular respiration in the tissues that combines oxygen and
        glucose to produce adenosine triphosphate (ATP) energy for cellular process
        and carbon dioxide as a by-product. When the demand for oxygen exceeds
        the supply then *anaerobic* respiration can be used to generate ATP energy;
        lactic acid is the by-product.

B3. Circulatory system

a) Heart and lungs

Deoxygenated blood from the venous system reaches the *right atrium* of the heart
from the body via the inferior and superior *vena cava*; it passes through the *tricuspid
valve* (contains three cusps/flaps) into the *right ventricle* of the heart to be pumped
out of the heart through the pulmonary *valve* (prevents backflow) via the *pulmonary
arteries* (the only artery to carry de-oxygenated blood) to the lungs; oxygenated blood
leaves the lungs via the *pulmonary veins* and reaches the *left atrium* of the heart,
passing through the *bicuspid* (mitral) *valve* and into the *left ventricle* before being
pumped out of the heart through the *aortic valve* into the *aorta* and to the body.

i)   Direction of flow: blood flows from the right to the left side of the heart via the
        lungs to be oxygenated: right atrium; tricuspid valve; right ventricle; pulmonary
        valve; pulmonary arteries (de-oxygenated); lungs; pulmonary capillaries
        (carbon dioxide lost and oxygen gained) pulmonary veins (oxygenated);
        bicuspid (mitral) valve; left ventricle; aortic valve; aorta and systemic arteries.

ii)   Order of valves (four) tricuspid, pulmonary, bicuspid (mitral), then aortic
        ('tricycle before bicycle').

iii)   Heart beat: rate controlled by electrical impulses from the sinoatrial (SA) node
        (pacemaker cells in the wall of the right atrium); atria contract first followed by
        the ventricles (impulses from the atrioventricular (AV) node, the bundle of His
        (AV bundle) and the Purkinje fibres); in other words, both atria contract together
        followed by both ventricles together a fraction of a second later.

iv)   Blood pressure: systolic over diastolic (eg 120/70): systole (heart contracts)
        and diastole (heart relaxes); systole + diastole = cardiac cycle
        (eg 75 cycles/min or one every 0.8 seconds).

v)   Cardiac output (ml/min) = stroke volume (ml) × heart rate (beats per minute).

b) Blood

i) Composition: 55% = plasma (of which 90% = water; 7% = proteins); 45% = cells (99% = red; 1% = white).

ii) Functions: transports oxygen, carbon dioxide, nutrients, waste products and hormones and clotting factors (plasma); regulates pH, temperature and osmotic pressure (plasma proteins); protects: *leucocytes* (white blood cells) fight infection; *lymphocytes* (two types): helper T-cells that mature in the thymus gland and B-cells that mature in the bone marrow and produce antibodies that respond to antigens (foreign bodies).

B4. Nervous system; eye

a) CNS and PNS

The central nervous system (CNS) includes the brain and spinal cord but excludes the peripheral nervous system (PNS). Thirty-one pairs of spinal nerves (left and right) fan out from the spinal cord to form the PNS.

i) Nerve impulse path: sensory *receptor* stimulated (eg skin), nerve impulses (electrical messages) sent via a sensory (*afferent*) neurone (ascending pathway) of the peripheral nervous system (PNS) to the central nervous system (CNS) and then away (descending pathway) from the CNS via a motor (*efferent*) neurone (of the PNS) to an *effector* (muscle or gland).

ii) Reflex arc: sensory receptor neurone stimulated (eg hot surface); nerve impulse sent via an afferent neurone to a motor neurone via an *interneurone* (a relay neurone) in the spinal cord (the brain receives an impulse later). The *cerebral cortex* can override the reflex arc (eg not wishing to drop a valuable hot object).

b) Autonomic (involuntary) nervous system (ANS)

Controls the automatic functions of the body that maintain stable internal conditions (ie *homeostasis*) (eg respiration, heart rate, blood pressure, temperature and salt-water balance). The *hypothalamus* (of the brain) regulates many of the body's autonomic systems (eg temperature through vasodilation/constriction; the *pons* regulates breathing).

c) The eye

The iris (two sets of muscles) controls the amount of light entering the pupil by contracting the circular muscle (for bright light) or the radial muscle (in dim light); the dilation or constriction of the pupil is by autonomic reflex arc. Photoreceptors (light-sensitive rod and cone cells), contained in the retina, measure intensity, wavelength and position of light; impulses are relayed via ganglion cells to the optic nerve, which transmits impulses to the brain. The image on the retina is inverted and results from the refraction of light at the cornea with fine adjustment at the lens; the image is sharpest near to the centre of the retina at the *fovea*. The focus of the lens can be altered from infinity (parallel light) to a near object by the *accommodation* reflex (focus at a near object = maximum accommodation = maximum curvature (more spherical)) (see also Physics P16f). The ciliary muscles are responsible for changing the shape of the lens: near object = ciliary muscles contract = suspensory ligaments loose = more convex lens (fatter) = more diffraction; distant object = ciliary muscles relaxed = suspensory ligaments taut = less convex lens (thinner) = less diffraction.

B5. Endocrine system; menstrual cycle hormones

a) Endocrine glands

Secrete *hormones* (chemical messengers) into the bloodstream; respond more slowly than the nervous system and the effects are longer-lasting.

i)   Pineal gland (*melatonin*) and pituitary gland (eg *growth hormone*; *oxytocin* in childbirth); thyroid (eg *thyroxine* to increase the metabolic rate) and parathyroid glands (eg increase blood calcium); thymus gland (*thymosin* for T-lymphocytes in immunity).

ii) Pancreas (eg *insulin* to reduce blood glucose levels and *glucagon* to increase blood sugar levels).

iii) Adrenal glands (eg *steroid hormones* in response to stress); ovaries (*oestrogen* and *progesterone*) and testes (*testosterone*). The kidney is not an endocrine gland but it secretes the hormone *erythropoietin* (EPO) to increase red blood cell production.

b) Negative feedback

Resists change; inhibits any deviation from the *norm*. Detection of a change inhibits the change; for example, food intake = a rise in blood glucose above the norm is detected by receptors in the pancreas = insulin hormone secreted by the pancreas (beta cells) travels to the *target organ* = liver stores glucose as glycogen = drop in blood glucose level = pancreas detects the drop and stops producing insulin = normal glucose levels achieved. If the blood glucose level is too low, the pancreas detects this and secretes glucagons (alpha cells), stimulating the release of glucose by the liver. Most homeostatic controls use negative feedback mechanism to *oppose any change*.

c) Positive feedback

Magnifies change; promotes any deviation from the norm.

Detection of a change stimulates the change, eg start of menstrual cycle = rise in pituitary FSH (follicle-stimulating hormone) = ovaries produce more oestrogen = rise in pituitary LH (luteinizing hormone) = ovaries produce more oestrogen = LH surge. A positive feedback mechanism *magnifies any change*.

d) Menstrual cycle hormones

FSH level rises promoting the growth of ovarian follicles that release *oestrogen*, causing the *endometrium* to build to full thickness; LH (luteinizing hormone) peaks on mid-cycle (day 14) to stimulate ovulation, that is, the release of a matured *oocyte* (egg) from the follicle into the Fallopian tube; LH acts on the empty follicle to form the *corpus luteum*, which secretes oestrogen and progesterone; the latter rises to maintain gestation and inhibit FSH (prevents further ovulation). If the egg is not fertilized with a sperm (ie no *zygote*) then the corpus luteum breaks down. Both positive and negative feedback loops operate during the menstrual cycle.

B6. Urinary system

a) Components

Kidneys, ureters, urinary bladder and urethra.

b) Kidney and nephron

i)   Kidney anatomy: renal cortex (outer), medulla (middle) and renal pelvis (inner) continuous with the ureter that leads into the bladder. *Nephrons* are the functional units of the kidney and extend from the cortex (glomerular filtration) into the medulla (filtrate re-absorption and urine concentration).

ii) Nephron: a schematic diagram of a nephron follows.

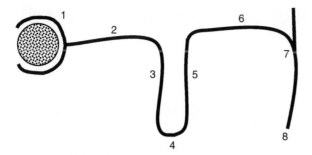

(1) *Renal corpuscle* = *Bowman's* capsule (glomerular capsule) + *glomerulus* (bundle of capillaries) attached to (2) the *proximal convoluted* (coiled) *tubule,* which leads into (3) the descending limb of (4) the *loop of Henle* (nephron loop or medullary loop), leading to (5) the ascending limb extending to (6) the *distal convoluted tubule* emptying into (7) the collecting duct and (8) the renal pelvis.

c) Filtration and selective re-absorption

1 = *Protein* not filtered out and remains in the blood.

2 = 100 per cent of *glucose* re-absorbed back into the blood capillaries; two-thirds of *sodium* (salt) and *water* re-absorbed.

3 = Only water is re-absorbed and not sodium.

4 = Sodium concentration is at its highest.

5 = Only sodium re-absorbed (eg pumped out when *aldosterone* is released by the endocrine gland on the top of each kidney).

6 = More sodium reabsorbed.

7 = If dehydrated (high *osmotic pressure*/solutes) antidiuretic hormone (ADH) is released by the pituitary gland and water is re-absorbed, otherwise urine remains dilute.

8 = Waste products excreted in urine: *urea* (50% of it) and creatinine (100% of it).

d) Blood flow

Aorta, renal artery, arteries of kidney; afferent arterioles to glomerulus capillaries; efferent arteriole from glomerulus to network of blood capillaries surrounding nephrons; veins of kidney, renal vein and inferior vena cava.

B7. DNA (deoxyribonucleic acid), genes and cell division

a) Genes

The nucleus of human cells contains 46 chromosomes (22 pairs and two sex chromosomes). Each chromosome contains thousands of genes made up of chains of DNA nucleotides. The nucleotides consist of a sugar molecule (deoxyribose), a phosphate group and one of four possible nitrogenous 'base pairs': adenine (A), cytosine (C), guanine (G) and thymine (T). Each rung in the DNA double-stranded helix ladder is an A to T or C to G base pair.

b) Gametes, somatic cells and the cell cycle

i) Gametes: diploid egg and sperm cells precursor cells divide by meiosis to produce male and female haploid *gametes* with nuclei that contain 23 chromosomes. These fuse during egg fertilization to produce a new cell, the *zygote*, which has a single diploid nucleus. During meiosis, diploid cells divide twice: once to give two diploid cells (DNA duplicated) and then once more to give four different haploid cells, each with a single copy of each chromosome (creates genetic variability); after fertilization the diploid chromosome number is restored. Only haploid cells, produced by meiosis and containing half the number of chromosomes, are suitable to become gametes.

ii) Somatic cells: these are non-sex cells that replicate by mitosis to produce two identical, diploid daughter cells with the same number of chromosomes as all the other somatic cells, including the zygote from which they originate.

iii) Cell cycle: cell growth and DNA replication (*interphase*) is followed by mitosis in four phases: *prophase* (chromosomes visible in nucleus and nuclear membrane dissolves), *metaphase* (line up along equator), *anaphase* (chromosomes move apart) and finally *telophase* (nuclear membranes form and the cell divides in two).

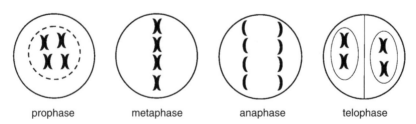

prophase   metaphase   anaphase   telophase

In other words, a cell can divide mitotically once it has two complete copies of its DNA (two copies from the father and two copies from the mother = ie $46 \times 2 = 92$ chromosomes after prophase).

B8. Patterns of inheritance

a) Punnett square

This shows all the possible combination of *alleles* derived from each parent; they can be either dominant (common) or recessive (rare); two alleles = one *genotype* (the DNA gentic code). The *phenotype* (trait) is the physical characteristic (eg brown eyes or blue eyes) expressed from the genotype. Thus: cells = nuclei = DNA = genes = alleles = genotypes = phenotypes (inherited *trait*).

b) Homozygous and heterozygous

i)   Two alleles the same = *homozygous* genotype; two different alleles = *heterozygous* genotype.

ii)   Dominant and recessive: two dominant alleles = *homozygous dominant*; two recessive alleles = *homozygous recessive*. One dominant allele and one recessive allele = *heterozygous* dominant (recessive allele is masked by the dominant one).

c) Inherited abnormalities/disease

Autosomal (22 matching pairs of non-sex chromosomes or autosomes) and *X-linked* (1 pair of sex chromosomes X and Y).

i)   **Autosomal dominant:** abnormality is in the dominant allele, eg Huntington's. If D = dominant trait (abnormality), d = recessive trait (normal) then heterozygous (Dd) will be abnormal; homozygous for the affected allele (DD) will be abnormal; homozygous for the normal allele (dd) will be normal. *Dominant genes (whether homozygous or heterozygous) always express the phenotype (= abnormality).*
Punnett squares: one homozygous affected parent (DD) = 100% affected children (all Dd); one heterozygous affected parent (Dd) = 50% affected children (50/50 Dd/dd). Punnett squares = DD × dd = Dd, Dd, Dd, Dd (100%) and Dd × dd = Dd, Dd, dd, dd (50/50) respectively.

ii) **Autosomal recessive:** abnormality is in the recessive allele, eg cystic fibrosis. If N = dominant trait (normal); n = recessive trait (genetic disease/abnormality), then heterozygous child (Nn) will be normal but a *carrier* for the affected gene; homozygous child for the normal allele (NN) will be normal; homozygous child for the affected allele (nn) will be abnormal. *Recessive genes must be homozygous if they are expressed in the phenotype; if heterozygous, a carrier.* Punnett squares: one homozygous affected parent (nn) × one homozygous unaffected parent (NN) = 100% of children are carriers (all Nn); one homozygous affected parent (nn) × one heterozygous unaffected parent (Nn; *carrier*) = 50% of children are carriers (Nn) and 50% affected (nn); two heterozygous parents (both Nn) = 50% carriers (Nn), 25% affected (nn), 25% unaffected (NN). Punnett squares = Nn, Nn, Nn, Nn (100%) and Nn, Nn, nn, nn (50/50). In the case of Nn, Nn, nn, NN (50/25/25), then in children not expressing the phenotype (ie Nn, Nn, NN), the probability of being a carrier (Nn) is two-thirds and the probability of not being a carrier (NN) is one-third.

iii) **X-linked inheritance:** abnormality/disease is caused by genes located on the X-chromosome; examples include haemophilia and colour blindness. Males are XY and females are XX. A male must pass his Y-gene on to his sons and his X-gene on to his daughters, so if he has the disease then all his daughters will inherit the affected gene but none of his sons. Affected females have a 50% chance that each son and each daughter will inherit the affected gene.

X-linked recessive X^a (most common): an affected male cannot have X-affected sons but his daughters are all carriers (they have a 'working copy' of the X-gene and do not develop the condition); female carriers have a 50% chance of a son being affected and a 50% chance of a daughter being a carrier. *X-linked abnormalities are passed on by female carriers and by affected males.*

X-linked dominant X^A (rare): affected male cannot have any X-affected sons (as per recessive) but his daughters are all affected; affected females have a 50% chance of a son being affected and a 50% chance of a daughter being affected (ie not a carrier). *If an affected male has an affected mother then she must be dominant for the trait; if the mother is not affected then she must be a carrier.*

d) Pedigree chart

Shows the genetic history of a family (eg grandparents, parents, children), that is, the inherited phenotypes. General patterns are as follows:

i)   Mostly males affected = X-linked abnormality.

ii)   Males and females affected equally = autosomal.

iii) Every generation affected = dominant for the abnormality.

iv)   Skips one or more generations = recessive for the abnormality.

For example, three generations: unaffected grandfather/grandmother with one married, affected son, one unaffected son, two unaffected daughters, one with affected sons.

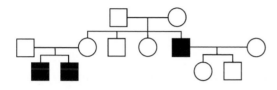

Key: male □ ; female ○ ; affected = shaded

X-linked recessive inheritance
(female carriers (heterozygous X^AX^a); males cannot pass on
the trait to their sons)

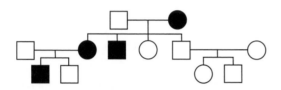

Key: male □ ; female ○ ; affected = shaded

X-linked dominant inheritance
(affected males have affected mother)

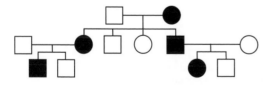

Key: male □ ; female ○ ; affected = shaded

Autosomal dominant inheritance (50% of males and 50% of females affected in
every generation with one affected parent (heterozygous))

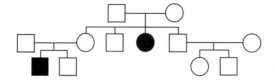

Key: male □ ; female ○ ; affected = shaded

Autosomal recessive (25% of the children of unaffected parents (heterozygous) will express the recessive trait (homozygous))

Biology review questions

Q1 (B8(1)) If two heterozygous, phenotypically tall plants with a recessive gene for height are cross-pollinated, what will be the ratio of tall plants to short in the offspring?

A. 1:1

B. 1:2

C. 2:1

D. 3:1

E. 4:1

Answer _____

Q2 (B8(3)) If A = dominant abnormal trait, a = recessive normal trait, B = dominant normal trait and b = recessive abnormal trait, then what genotypes are expressed in the following pedigree?

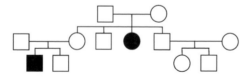

Key: male □ ; female ○ ; affected = shaded

Autosomal recessive (25% of the children of unaffected parents (heterozygous) will express the recessive trait (homozygous))

A. aa, Bb

B. Bb, bb

C. Bb, Bb

D. BB, Bb

Answer _____

Q3   (B8(3)) If A = dominant abnormal trait, a = recessive normal trait, B = dominant normal trait and b = recessive abnormal trait, then what genotypes are expressed in the following pedigree?

A. AA, Aa, aa
B. AA, aa
C. Aa, Aa
D. AA, aa, bb

Answer [   ]

Q4   (B4) Choose the correct word or term (labelled A to K) from the list below to match each numbered space (i to vii) in the text below. Some words or terms may be used more than once or not at all.

A = ascending; B = constrict; C = close; D = distant; E = autonomic; F = ciliary; G = rods and cones; H = convex; I = concave; J = optic nerve; K = efferent.

The iris of the eye acts as its aperture and is a good example of an [...i...] reflex. Light enters via the pupil and stimulates the [...ii...] in the retina. Impulses are sent to the central nervous system via the [...iii...]. The oculomotor nerve in the [...iv...] limb of the reflex arc innervates the muscles of the iris, controlling the size of the pupil. In the 'accommodation' reflex the [...v...] muscles adjust the focus of the lens. Long-sighted people can only see [...vi...] objects clearly and need glasses with a [...vii...] lens to refract the light more.

i   = ...
ii = ...
iii = ...
iv = ...
v   = ...
vi = ...
vii = ...

Q5   (B5c,d) In the menstrual cycle, which hormone peaks to trigger ovulation and which hormone peaks after ovulation has taken place?

A. Oestrogen followed by progesterone.
B. Follicle-stimulating hormone followed by progesterone.
C. Luteinizing hormone followed by progesterone.
D. Follicle-stimulating hormone followed by luteinizing hormone.
E. Luteinizing hormone followed by oestrogen.

Answer [   ]

Q6   (B1) Most of the chemical digestion of carbohydrates, protein and fats takes place in which part of the gastro-intestinal tract catalysed by enzymes released by which gland(s)?

A. Stomach and thyroid gland.
B. Stomach and pancreas gland.
C. Duodenum and adrenal glands.
D. Small intestine and pancreas gland.
E. Small intestine and pituitary gland.

Answer [   ]

Q7   (B8(1)) In the Punnett square shown below, 'A' is the dominant allele and 'a' is the recessive allele. How many genotypes are there and how many phenotypes are there?

	A	a
A	AA	Aa
a	Aa	aa

A. 2 genotypes and 2 phenotypes.
B. 3 genotypes and 2 phenotypes.
C. 2 genotypes and 3 phenotypes.
D. 3 genotypes and 3 phenotypes.
E. 3 genotypes and 4 phenotypes.

Answer [   ]

Q8   (B2b, 3a) Red blood cells (RBCs) in the pulmonary artery contain:

A. Less carbon dioxide than RBCs in the pulmonary vein and no oxygen.
B. Less oxygen than RBCs in the pulmonary vein and no carbon dioxide.
C. Less oxygen and less carbon dioxide than RBCs in the pulmonary vein.
D. More oxygen and more carbon dioxide than RBCs in the pulmonary vein.
E. Less oxygen and more carbon dioxide than RBCs in the pulmonary vein.

Answer

Q9   (B6) Which of the following substances are not found in the glomerular filtrate of a healthy kidney nephron?

1: urea; 2: glucose; 3: protein; 4: water; 5: sodium; 6: red blood cells.

A. 1, 2, 4 and 5
B. 2, 4 and 5
C. 3 and 6
D. 1 and 3
E. 2, 3 and 6

Answer

CHAPTER 6

Writing task review

In the BMAT writing task you have to answer one question out of the three choices available. The questions typically relate to philosophical or socio-cultural issues, which may favour candidates with an A level in the humanities. There is a time limit of 30 minutes and you can write no more than one A4 side of text, or about 300 words. If your handwriting is small or condensed you might exceed 350 words but if it is large or spaced out then you might only manage 270. Either way, most people, writing a minimum speed of 20 words per minute, will be able to write their answer in under 15 minutes, leaving 10 minutes to prepare the essay with a few minutes to check through it at the end.

W1. Choice of question (1 minute)

Read through *all* three questions quickly but carefully before making a decision. Grade each question after you have read it. If you like the question then give it a tick; if you are uncertain but it seems possible then give it a question mark; if it is definitely not the question for you then give it a cross. Do not assume automatically that the question you have ticked is the best choice. Look again at the more challenging question; it may offer the better-prepared candidate the chance to excel. NB: before you make your final decision, make sure that you can see *both sides of the argument*.

W2. Preparation (10 minutes)

Thorough planning is an essential part of your answer. It needs a beginning, middle and an end that cover all parts of the question. This hints at three paragraphs; however, an additional paragraph at the start serves as an introduction when the questions ask you to explain what you think the author means or is trying to imply.

i) **Paragraphs:** each paragraph informs the examiner that you are covering a new aspect of the question, and each sentence in the paragraph carries a single idea related to the theme of the paragraph.

ii) **Sentences:** your sentences can (and should) vary in length from the short, for example 15 words or less, to the long, for example 26 words or more. Shorter sentences are easy to read and understand but if there are too many they make your work sound choppy and your ideas fragmented. Longer sentences make your ideas sound *unified* but they are more difficult to read and if a sentence carries too much detail the meaning becomes obscure. By way of example, the sentences on this page average 24 words.

iii) **Layout:** taking an average sentence length of 24 words, then you will need to write about 13 sentences in four paragraphs. By way of example, you could use a 2,3,4,4-sentence plan, consisting of two sentences for the introduction; three arguments that support the statement, including one example; four arguments that counter it, including one example; followed by a four-sentence conclusion.

W3. The four-paragraph approach (10 minutes preparation)

Four paragraphs: introduction, arguments for, arguments against and conclusion. Each paragraph relates to one aspect of this approach.

i) **First paragraph** (eg two sentences): at the preparatory stage you need to *identify the task* and jot down what it entails. The introduction usually involves paraphrasing, that is, re-stating in *your own words* what the question is asking or what points the author is trying to make. If the question contains a hidden assumption (see section A1b) then you may wish to highlight it here, but not to excess. Explain what the statement means to you in two or three sentences at most.

ii) **Second and third paragraphs:** use *brainstorming* as a first step to generate any ideas without judging their value; it is the quantity rather than the quality of the ideas that matters at this stage. Even so, it is worth classifying the ideas as either for or against the argument. You can do this by placing key words or phrases in two opposing columns, for or against the argument/statement.

FOR (eg choose your three best ideas in support of the argument)	AGAINST (eg choose your four best ideas counter to the argument)
Hints and tips when choosing ideas:	Hints and tips when choosing ideas:
• Avoid including too many examples; one may suffice. An example is not a substitute for a well-crafted argument. • Do not leave your best ideas until the last in an attempt to build a crescendo. Get to the heart of the matter straight away; you have 20 minutes. • Use arrows to link brainstorming ideas that are counter to each other.	• Avoid including too many examples; one or two examples that counter the argument may suffice. • Do not get drawn into an emotional response even if you disagree strongly with what is being asserted. Be dispassionate; do not set yourself against the argument. Maintain a balanced view and avoid unnecessary bias.

iii) **Fourth paragraph:** *Evaluate and synthesize* your arguments (discuss strengths and weaknesses) to formulate a coherent conclusion that takes a clear position or reconciles the differences (you can introduce your own opinions).

W4. Composing the essay (15 minutes)

Points to remember:

i)   Do not deviate from your chosen topic and answer all the components.
      Make a confident start, for example:

   – 'I believe that the statement implies that…'
   – 'The statement argues that…'
   – 'The author makes the point that…'

ii)   Remember to keep your handwriting legible.

iii) Be careful with your grammar, spelling and syntax to avoid losing marks.
      Avoid jargon or abbreviations. If you were to use the word 'cerebrovascular accident', put CVA in brackets after it; now you can use CVA if you need it

again. Alternatively you could use the word 'stroke' as no special technical knowledge is expected.

iv) Follow your plan, keeping to one theme per paragraph; use linking words and phrases to facilitate a smooth transition from one paragraph to the next and to inform the examiner that you are starting a new theme, for example:

- 'On the other hand…'
- 'To counter these assertions…'
- 'However, it might also be said…'

v) Vary the length of your sentences whilst keeping to one idea per sentence; short sentences make your work easier to understand.

vi) Use bullet points or roman numerals to make sequential points clearly (as in this list) but you must write a *unified* essay.

vii) The final paragraph: here you can take a clear position as long as you have weighed up the arguments for and against to reach an informed decision.

W5. Sources and resources

Preparing for the essay section of the BMAT requires a far more diverse selection of resources than the other sections. Imagine you have a title as follows:

'A cost to an individual can be justified by a benefit to the group.'

What sources of examples might you come up with? Try thinking about the following categories:

i)   Medical

ii) Scientific (not specifically medical)

iii) Arts, humanities, politics and law

It will be useful to incorporate a mix of ideas coming from each of the different categories, to demonstrate your understanding of medicine, scientific acumen and breadth of knowledge.

For example, for the above question you may wish to consider:

i)   Medical

'An example in favour of the author's statement can be of a medical trial testing a new drug. Usually, during the medical trials two groups of patients are used: one group is given a real drug and another is given a placebo. Also, a double-blind

technique might be used, which means that neither the patient nor the prescriber knows which drug is given to avoid bias in an experiment.

Sometimes, when a new drug is considered to be successful, the patient who was prescribed a placebo will feel no improvement and might even die, but those patients who were taking a real drug will either have their disease cured or at least make some improvement. In this case, the author of the quote is right to say that a cost to an individual, who, perhaps, would remain ill, suffer or even die anyway, can be justified by a benefit to the group, because, as a result of a successful trial a new effective drug that will save the lives of a great deal of people might be produced.'

Notice how the student demonstrates her knowledge of a key medical concept, the double-blinded placebo controlled trial, but applies it directly to the question.

ii)   Scientific

'Space exploration by humans has carried some risk to the brave astronauts, and 18 individuals have lost their lives in all manned space flights. Technical failures, fires and even adverse weather on landing have resulted in these incidents. This amounts to approximately five per cent of individuals who have launched, and of course the cost to these individuals is immeasurable. However, this cost to individuals who participate of their own free will, with knowledge and understanding of the risks and some compensation in terms of their payment, might be considered to be justified by furthering mankind's knowledge about the universe. In extremis, since the Sun will one day expand to a red giant and consume the earth, if their first steps into space were never taken, the human race might never escape this fate. Even with the cost to themselves, the benefit to mankind as a species may yet be justified, even if it isn't quite yet.'

The student moves on to use an example of science which is not directly related to medicine, again demonstrating her grasp of, and interest and passion for physics, but tempering it again directly and provocatively to the question.

iii) Arts, humanities, politics and law

'The nuclear bombardment of Hiroshima and Nagasaki in 1945 is an example against the author's quote. Two innocent cities were sacrificed in order to make Japan surrender in the Second World War. In this case, it is difficult to assess if the cost to the individuals who died can be justified by the benefit of those who were saved by rapidly ending the war. One could attempt to calculate the numbers, based on the rate of progress the allied forces were making towards key targets in Japan, and project the cost in lives on previous data. However, to some people the qualitative fact of the indiscriminate killing of non-combatants cannot be justified.'

In this example, the student is showing her range of knowledge, and drawing upon examples outside of pure science. Notice how she does not force her own position into the example but states that some may find this event unjustifiable, again directing things back to the title.

There can be some crossover in these categories, for example if the student referred to the infamous Tuskagee Siphilis Experiment, where African-Americans were deliberately given syphilis and never treated for it or informed of its treatment. This trial started in 1932 in the USA. This is a good example of biomedical research which was considered highly unethical, but also demonstrates historical knowledge and interest.

As you can see, the range of sources and resources must be broad to allow you to give a well rounded answer. Consider the use of the following:

i)   Medical

Medical journals, medical and health sections of newspapers are traditional sources. Online blogs and videos, particularly those by clinicians and healthcare workers, can be useful. Make sure you include some sources from doctors who face adverse conditions, such as those working for MSF or the International Red Cross, as well as those who have faced disciplinary hearings with the GMC.

ii) Scientific (not specifically medical)

New Scientist, other general scientific magazines and textbooks are traditional sources. You may find it helpful to include some historical examples of scientific discoveries, in which case 'history of science' books and websites will be of interest.

iii) Arts, humanities, politics and law

Since you will already be busy preparing for the other BMAT sections, you cannot possibly learn everything there is to know. Make it count, and make it sustainable, by following subjects you might be interested in. Any subject from literature to classics, economics to law can be drawn upon. Make sure that you are writing brief notes on anything useful you might read: you never want to revisit the core text and read it over again.

W6. The final check (2–3 minutes)

Spend a few minutes reading through your essay to check your punctuation, spelling and grammar, and to spot any missed-out words. Have you avoided repetition? Does it flow with good transitions between paragraphs? Remember your answer must not exceed a single side of A4 paper.

Example essay 1. Patients should not be offered choices in their medical treatment; doctors know what is best for them

What does the author mean by this statement? Develop a counter-argument. Do you believe that patients should be allowed to choose their own treatments?

For	Against
1. Patient expects doctor to find a cure.	1. Patient autonomy; the right to choose.
2. Doctor more knowledgeable, also impartial/objective.	2. Patient not involved = poor self-care, eg diabetes.
3. Doctor knows the best treatment options.	3. Doctor's choice may not suit the individual's needs.
	4. Doctor takes all of the responsibility.

Essay 1

The author believes that doctors are the best people to make decisions about a patient's treatment.[1] The statement implies that patients can be excluded from the decision-making process.[2]

Whilst the author's view is very one-sided, it is true that patients look to their doctor to diagnose health problems and offer curative treatments [*supports argument*].[3] Furthermore, [*more support*] patients may lack the necessary knowledge to make decisions about their treatment and are not best placed to view their health problems impartially or dispassionately.[4]

However [*against*], it is not appropriate for a doctor to dictate to a patient what should and should not be done to the patient's own body.[5] This would be ethically unsound as it detracts from freedom of choice and might infringe upon the patient's human rights.[6] In addition [*also against*], unless the patient is involved in the decision-making process, the outcome of the treatment may not meet with the patient's lifestyle needs.[7] For example, [*one only*] failure to discuss treatments for diabetes may lead to poor patient practices in blood sugar control; errors in self-injecting insulin, for example, could be dangerous.[8] Furthermore, [*against again*] should a treatment fail, the patient will blame the doctor for the poor outcome and will not share any of the responsibility.[9]

> Although it is beneficial for patients to be included in the decision-making process, this is not to say that they should dictate their treatments [*last part of question*].[10] The NHS is a rationed service that has to meet the needs of patients fairly within the resources available.[11] Thus [*reconciling*], whilst some patients may wish to remain as passive recipients in their medical treatment, ideally all patients should be included in the decision-making process.[12] The doctor should discuss the treatment options with the patient to facilitate joint decisions that satisfy both parties.[13]

The following example essay also uses a four-paragraph approach but does so in a different way. The arguments supporting the statement flow naturally from the introduction and an additional paragraph is used to answer the second part of the question.

Example essay 2. Mental health has nothing to do with physical well-being

What do you take this statement to mean? Develop a counter-argument that refutes the author's view. Do you believe that a healthy mind equals a healthy body?

For	Against
1. Can be physically healthy and mentally ill at same time.	1. Mental illness: loss of motivation to maintain health; self-neglect.
2. Psychiatric medicine is a distinct branch of medicine.	2. Illness = physical stress = mental stress. = mental illness
3. Physical ailments do not lead to mental health problems.	3. Pain; anxiety; eg heart attack leads to depression.
	4. Positive mental attitude is good for recovery.

Essay 2

The statement implies that there is no synergy between the mind and the body where mental and physical health is concerned. It also suggests that mental illness cannot be blamed on a lack of physical health. The fact that the treatment of psychiatric problems is a separate branch of medicine may lend support to this view. Furthermore, [*more support*] it is certainly the case that a person can be mentally ill yet physically healthy at the same time.

However, [*against*] people who suffer from mental health problems may be less motivated to maintain their physical health or may lack the capacity to do so. For example, [*first one*] lack of mental health can detract from physical health when a person fails to hold down a job and a lack of money leads to a poor diet or bad housing. More directly, [*second example*] stress and anxiety can lead to a rise in blood pressure, which increases the risk of heart disease and stroke; physical illness and the experience of hospitalization can be highly stressful.

Whilst it may be difficult to show empirically [*measure*] that a healthy mind equals a healthy body, [*second part of question*] people with a positive outlook on life are more likely to adopt healthier lifestyles. It is generally accepted that a positive mental attitude towards physical illness speeds recovery. By way of example, the prevention of depression in heart attack patients increases their chances of regaining health and reduces mortality.

It is clear that the experience of physical illness and the failure to cope with it can be detrimental to mental health and that mental health problems can, either directly or indirectly, impair physical health. However, [*reconciling*] it is also true that a healthy body does not guarantee a healthy mind any more than a healthy mind can guarantee a healthy body.

The following tests should be attempted under exam conditions as per the BMAT: that is, in the allotted time and without a calculator or dictionary. These are full mock tests and provide the equivalent of three BMAT tests (nine papers). Candidates will find some questions easier than others, depending upon their chosen college subjects.

Almost every question comes with its revision topics shown in parentheses. For example (P3b; M6d) means revise Physics topic 3b and Maths topic 6d; (B1a; C10b,c) means revise Biology topic 1a and Chemistry topics 10b and 10c. The mock tests in this book are regarded as part of the learning process, and for this reason some questions include a helpful hint as to the method of solution. These hints encourage you to have a go rather than to jump to the answer if you feel you cannot do it. However, candidates should try to answer the question without referring to the hint in the first instance.

BMAT SECTION 1 (Mock tests 1, 4 and 7): Aptitude and skills

You have 35 questions to answer in one hour. Calculators are not permitted. Record your answers on a separate sheet of paper.

BMAT SECTION 2 (Mock tests 2, 5 and 8): Scientific knowledge and applications

You have 30 minutes to answer 27 questions. Calculators are not permitted. Record your answers on a separate sheet of paper.

BMAT SECTION 3 (Mock test 3, 6 and 9): Writing task

You have 30 minutes to write a unified essay on one of the questions. Your answer must be contained on a single side of A4 paper (30 lines). Dictionaries are not permitted.

PART TWO

Tests and answers

CHAPTER 7

Mock tests

Section 1 Aptitude and skills

Mock test 1

35 questions
Time allowed one hour
No calculators

Q1 (A2, 3) Motorway speed limits should no longer be restricted to 70 mph. More than half of all motorists admit to driving at 80 mph or above so it may as well be made legal. Driving at 10 mph above the current limit is not frowned upon and few drivers believe that they will be prosecuted for doing so.

Which of the following best expresses the main point of the passage?

A. It is as safe to drive at 80 mph as it is at 70 mph.
B. Most drivers are quite happy to disobey speed limits.
C. Drivers frequently exceed 80 mph on motorways.
D. Driving at 80 mph on motorways is accepted behaviour.
E. Cars can be driven at 80 mph without fear of prosecution.

Answer ☐

Q2   (A2, 3) Non-smokers should take priority over smokers where NHS treatment is concerned. People who engage in smoking are responsible for their own health problems. Those people who have made efforts to maintain their health should not have to wait for treatment behind smokers who have ignored it.

Statement: If all the non-smokers who failed to exercise, watch their weight or avoid excessive alcohol consumption went to the back of the queue there would be few people left at the front.

Which of the following best describes how the short statement relates to the argument?

A. It lends significant support to the argument.
B. It presents a significant challenge to the argument.
C. It restates the conclusion of the argument.
D. It restates one of the premises of the argument.
E. It neither supports nor challenges the argument.

Answer _____

Q3   (A2, 3) Nuclear power provides cheap and clean electricity. Almost 80 per cent of the electricity needs of France are met by nuclear power plants compared to a paltry 20 per cent in the UK. Coal-fired power stations produce 50 times more carbon dioxide per kilowatt-hour than do nuclear power plants, and fossil fuels will eventually run out. The government should support a new generation of nuclear power stations to tackle climate change and ensure sustainable energy supplies in the future. The UK lags behind France in nuclear technology so the power stations will have to be built and run by French companies.

Which one of the following, if true, would most seriously weaken the above argument?

A. The UK has a better spread of energy sources than France and can look towards 'renewables' for additional power.
B. The UK will lose its independence in power generation if nuclear power stations dominate energy sources.
C. The construction and decommissioning of nuclear reactors are expensive, and have a large carbon footprint.
D. Cutting back on energy consumption would reduce carbon dioxide emissions without the risks from nuclear power.
E. France's lack of natural resources meant that it had to embrace nuclear power.

Answer _____

Q4   (M9a) What fraction of the square is shaded if A and C are the mid-points of the two sides?

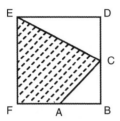

Answer [   ]

Q5   (M13b) The bar chart compares the hospital admissions for asthma per 100 000 population, for children in selected European countries. There are 12 million children in the UK and 10 million in Spain. How many children in the UK have been admitted to hospital with asthma?

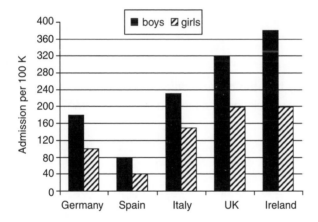

A.   24 000
B.   32 000
C.   52 000
D.   62 400
E.   84 000

Answer [   ]

Q6   (M13b) What is the difference between the UK and Spain in the number of hospital admissions for boys?

  A.   24 000
  B.   22 400
  C.   30 400
  D.   20 000
  E.   32 000

Answer

Q7   (M4b) What is the boy-to-girl ratio of hospital admissions in the UK, assuming the UK has an equal population of male and female children?

  A.   8:5
  B.   1:1.6
  C.   4:3
  D.   1:1
  E.   3:2

Answer

Q8   (M4b) Which country had the highest ratio of boys to girls, assuming each country has an equal population of male and female children?

  A.   Germany.
  B.   Spain.
  C.   Italy.
  D.   UK.
  E.   Ireland.

Answer

Q9   (A) Which shape comes next in the following sequence of shapes?

Answer

Q10 (A2, 3) Wind farms are a poor source of power. When the wind stops blowing, not a single watt of power is produced.

Which of the following is an implicit assumption of the above argument?

A. The wind must blow continuously for power to be produced.
B. Lack of wind makes wind farms an unreliable power source.
C. Wind farms can only produce power intermittently.
D. Wind farms are an expensive means of producing power.
E. Failure to produce power makes wind farms a poor power source.

Answer

Q11 (A2, 3) Cellulitis is a bacterial skin infection that mainly affects the extremities. It can be treated with anti-microbial therapy directed by blood culture and antibiotic sensitivity results. However, contamination by other bacteria on the skin usually leads to a high proportion of false positives.

Which of the following can safely be inferred from the above paragraph?

A. It is best to wait for the results of a blood culture and sensitivity test before initiating anti-microbial therapy.
B. Cellulitis will only respond to one antibiotic.
C. Bacterial contamination leads to a low proportion of false negatives.
D. The taking of blood cultures is often of no help in directing the treatment of cellulitis.
E. Cases of cellulitis are restricted to the arms and legs.

Answer

Q12 Place the following four sentences in the order in which they form the most coherent passage.

A. Deep sea organisms do not replenish their carbon from the air so they contain a higher proportion of inactive carbon.
B. Carbon-14 dating is not an infallible method of determining the age of ancient artefacts and organic matter.
C. Consequently they can have an anomalous carbon-dating age that appears much older than the true age.
D. It works best on once-living remains that consumed carbon from the air where the carbon-14 to carbon-12 ratio is fixed.

Answer

Q13 (A2, 3) In order to cause an infection, pathogenic bacteria must find a host. Therefore, if pathogenic bacteria find a host they will cause an infection.

To which one of the following criticisms is the above argument vulnerable?

A.   It assumes that all pathogenic bacteria will find a host.
B.   It assumes that finding a host is sufficient for pathogenic bacteria to cause an infection.
C.   It assumes that pathogenic bacteria cause infections.
D.   It assumes that after finding a host there is a high probability that the pathogenic bacteria will cause an infection.
E.   It assumes that pathogenic bacteria require a host to cause an infection.

Answer _____

Q14 (A2, 3) Cannabis should be legalized for both recreational and medicinal use. Marijuana is not considered addictive and smoking a 'joint' or 'reefer' is no different from smoking tobacco; its effects are similar to that of alcohol intoxication without the tendency for antisocial behaviour. Furthermore, the many and varied medical benefits of cannabis are well known. For example, the medical profession acknowledges that cannabis can relieve the symptoms of multiple sclerosis (MS). Therefore, the main reason for not legalizing cannabis must be the moral judgement that all drugs are bad; cannabis is a drug so cannabis is bad.

Which of the following is an unstated assumption of the above argument?

A.   Cannabis is less addictive than tobacco.
B.   Alcohol can lead to antisocial behaviour, unlike cannabis.
C.   Like all drugs, cannabis is bad.
D.   Cannabis use in MS is supported by the medical profession.
E.   There is no difference between recreational and medicinal use.

Answer _____

Q15 (M2e) Find the two missing numbers in the following series.

0, 1, 1, 2, 3, 5, ?, ?, 21, 34.

Answer _____

Q16 (M9) The diagram shows a square wedding cake iced on all sides excluding the base. It measures 30 cm × 30 cm × 15 cm deep. It is to be cut into identical portions measuring 5 cm × 5 cm × 5 cm. How many portions will have icing on them?

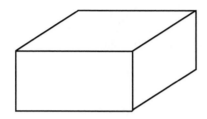

A.   90
B.   76
C.   60
D.   48
E.   40

(hint: 3 layers)

Answer

Q17 (M7b) A wholesaler buys a book from a publisher with a discount of 50 per cent off the retail price. The wholesaler marks the book up 40 per cent for the bookshop. What percentage does the bookseller add on to reach retail price? Give your answer to the nearest whole number.

Answer

Q18   (P5) The graph shows the speed of a train passing five stations: H, I, J, K and L.

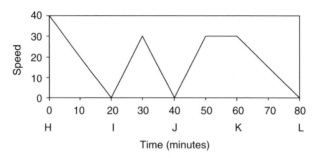

Which two pairs of stations are the same distances apart?

A.   HI and JK.
B.   HI and KL.
C.   IJ and KL.
D.   IJ and JK.
E.   HJ and JL.

Answer

Q19   If six guests at a dinner party all shake hands with each other, how many handshakes will there be?

A.   16
B.   15
C.   14
D.   12
E.   10

(hint: hexagon)

Answer

Q20 (M13a) The pie charts show the distribution of A-level grades in two different schools, X and Y.

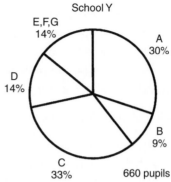

Which of the following can be deduced from the pie charts?

i.   School X achieved more A-grades at A level than School Y.
ii. The number of pupils achieving grade C or above in School X is 528.
iii. The A–C pass rate in School Y was 5 per cent above that in School X.

A. i and ii
B. ii and iii
C. i and iii
D. All
E. None

Answer [   ]

Q21 (A2, 3) People on low incomes cannot afford to eat a healthy diet. Instead they eat high-fat snack foods like chocolate, which contains more calories per unit cost than fresh fruit and vegetables.

Which of the following is the best statement of the flaw in the above argument?

A. Most people on low incomes are not undernourished.
B. Chocolate contains more calories but it is less satiating than fresh foods.
C. Meals containing fresh fruit and vegetable take too long to prepare in comparison with snack foods.
D. Most people on low incomes count cost but not calories when choosing food.

Answer [   ]

Q22 (A2, 3) Today, medical paternalism has given way to patient autonomy. This means that each individual has the right to accept, choose or refuse a treatment based on what each believes to be in his or her own best interests. Failure to consent to a life-saving treatment no longer implies that the patient is incapable of making the 'right decision'. Doctors have a duty to ensure that patients are able to make an informed choice, including why one course of treatment might be the preferred option, but they cannot exert any pressure beyond that of 'gentle persuasion'.

Which of the following best summarizes the passage?

A. The doctor should assist a patient in making decisions that are consistent with the patient's own beliefs and values.
B. The patient's viewpoint is the only one that is important when deciding upon a medical treatment.
C. The doctor must respect the patient's wishes at all times even when the patient's life is at risk.
D. The doctor must act in the patient's best interests by identifying the preferred treatment option.

Answer _____

Q23 (A2, 3). Pensioners account for one-fifth of the population and will need 75 per cent of their former earnings, amounting to 15 per cent of gross domestic product (GDP), if they are to avoid a sharp decline in living standards. The state pension amounts to a paltry 4 per cent of GDP and private pensions can barely match this meagre amount, leaving a large gap. Clearly many people of retirement age are going to find it hard to make ends meet in the future.

Which two of the following show that the conclusion is unsafe even if the evidence is correct?

A. It might be the case that many people of retirement age will choose to carry on working to make up the gap.
B. It might be that in the future GDP will increase, which means that pensions will also rise.
C. It might be the case that the stock market will improve and income from private pensions will increase twofold.
D. It might be the case that many pensioners will make ends meet on less than three-quarters of their former earnings.

Answer _____

Q24 (M13e) The table shows the percentage of females with a cardiovascular-related condition, by age and diagnosis.

Diagnosis/Age	25–34	35–44	45–54	55–64	65–74	75+
Angina	0.0	0.2	1.3	3.1	6.3	9.1
Heart murmur	1.0	0.9	1.2	1.4	1.8	2.2
Arrhythmia	1.0	1.5	2.2	2.5	3.3	4.2
Myocardial infarction	0.0	0.2	0.3	0.6	0.7	1.7
Stroke	0.1	0.1	0.1	0.3	0.4	1.8
Diabetes	0.3	0.9	1.5	2.5	4.8	5.3
Hypertension	1.5	3.7	7.8	20.5	27.9	26.8

Which conditions show more than a 500 per cent increase in prevalence between the age ranges of 45–54 and 75+?

A. Angina only.
B. Angina and myocardial infarction.
C. Angina, myocardial infarction and diabetes.
D. Angina, myocardial infarction and hypertension.
E. Angina, myocardial infarction and stroke.

Answer

Q25 (M12a.iv) The incidence of which conditions varies the least with age?

Answer

Q26 (A4b) If most members of a ramblers' group are members of a hikers' group and a few of the hikers are members of a climbers' group, then which of the following statements must be true?

i.   Most members of the climbers' group are not ramblers.
i.   Most members of the hikers' group are ramblers.
iii. No members belong to all three groups.

A. i only.
B. ii only.
C. iii only.
D. i and ii only.
E. none.

(hint: three-circle problem, C,R,H, left to right)

Answer

Q27 (A2) Consider the following two statements and the conclusion that follows:

    i)   Aptitude tests are a reliable predictor of degree performance (*major premise*).

    ii)   The BMAT is an aptitude test (*minor premise*).

    iii) The BMAT is a reliable predictor of degree performance (*conclusion*).

Which one of the following is invalid?

A.   If i) is false then iii) is unsafe.
B.   If ii) is false then iii) is unsafe.
C.   If iii) is true then i) and ii) are true.
D.   If iii) is unsafe then i) and/or ii) are false.
E.   If i) and ii) are true then iii) is safe.

Answer [＿＿＿＿＿]

Q28 (A2, 3) Global warming is good news for older people. Mortality rates are always higher in the winter than in the summer. Paradoxically, the wintertime 'excess mortality' in cold countries like Russia is lower than that of more moderate climates like the UK. People in cold countries are used to the cold and know more about keeping themselves warm than do people in temperate climates. However, the increasing prosperity of warmer countries helps to reduce winter deaths through reduced fuel poverty and people's ability to keep warm in their cars rather than having to rely on public transport.

Which two of the following can be concluded from the passage?

A.   The increased prosperity of warmer countries mitigates the effects of winter on their excess mortality rates.
B.   Global warming will reduce the winter excess mortality in Russia more than in the UK.
C.   The paradox is that the outdoor temperature is not the only factor affecting winter mortality rates.
D.   Both global warming and increasing prosperity will reduce excess mortality rates in the UK and Russia.
E.   The ratio of deaths in winter to deaths in summer is lower in Russia than in the UK.

Answer [＿＿＿＿＿]

Q29 (A2, 3) Calculators should be banned from school until after pupils have mastered mental arithmetic. It is essential that young people can solve arithmetic problems in their heads or on paper without having to resort to a calculator. In medical sciences, over-reliance on calculators has led to fatal 'order of magnitude' errors because practitioners lacked the mental agility to estimate the answer to a drug dosage calculation or identify a wrong answer.

Which one of the following, if true, would lend the greatest support to the above argument?

A. Drug dosage calculation errors reflect a lack of calculator proficiency rather than a lack of mental arithmetic skills.
B. Practitioners who pass a mental arithmetic test make fewer drug dosage errors than those who fail the test.
C. Over-reliance on calculators leads to over-confidence in drug dosage calculations.
D. Practitioners who use calculators are less likely to identify drug dosages that are 10 times greater than they should be.

Answer _____

Q30 (M13c) The graph below shows the approximate incidence of prostate cancer and colorectal cancer in men per million men, between 1980 and 1994.

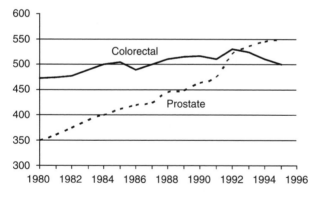

Reading from the graph, what was the average annual rate of increase in the incident rate of prostate cancer between 1984 and 1994 per million men?

A. 10
B. 13
C. 15
D. 18
E. 20

Answer _____

Q31 (M13c) If 10 000 men were diagnosed with colorectal cancer in 1995, how many men were in the population group?

    A.   10 million.
    B.   20 million.
    C.   25 million.
    D.   30 million.
    E.   1 million.

Answer [   ]

Q32 Carl is younger than Zak but older than Richard. Leanne is older than Carl but younger than Sarah. Which of the following statements cannot be true?

    A.   Richard is the youngest.
    B.   Zak is the oldest.
    C.   Sarah is the same age as Zak.
    D.   Carl is the second oldest.
    E.   Leanne is younger than Zak.

(hint: draw a young-to-old continuum line)

Answer [   ]

Q33 (M12b) A medical student sat two progress tests, T1 and T2. Each test was split into two sections, A and B, which were marked separately, and in the case of test T2 carried different weightings, as shown in the table. Calculate the combined percentage for the two tests (T1 and T2) if the marks for test T1 carry twice the weight of the marks for test T2.

	Test %		Weighting	
	A	B	A	B
Test T1	60%	72%	50%	50%
Test T2	90%	55%	40%	60%

(hint: per cent mark × decimal weight; add; 2/3, 1/3)

Answer [   ]

Questions 34 and 35 refer to the following information:

'Passing off' is a term used when a business attempts to mislead customers into believing that they are dealing with a well-known, more established business, through the use of confusingly similar trade marks or trade names. For example, McDonald's has taken legal action against several businesses that refused to drop Mc from their trading name, including those with phonetically similar names such as Macdonalds, Mcdonald, and Mcdonalds. The protection of a trading name is essential because associations with a lesser business can damage the reputation of an established business.

McDonald's has not always won its legal cases. However, it was more likely to succeed if the business had a clear association with a food service that could be confused with McDonald's. Thus, Elizabeth McCaughey was forced to change the name of her coffee shop from McCoffee and a Scottish sandwich shop owner had to change the name McMunchies, but McChina Wok Away was permitted because it was ruled that McChina would not cause any confusion amongst customers. It was also indicated that McDonald's did not have the right to the prefix Mc. Despite this ruling, McDonald's won its case against McCurry when a high court judge ruled that the use of the prefix Mc combined with colours distinctive of the McDonald's brand might confuse and deceive customers; the business had claimed that McCurry stood for Malaysian Chicken Curry.

Norman McDonald ran a small restaurant named McDonald's Hamburgers; Country drive-in. He fell foul of the McDonald's restaurant chain by including a couple of lit golden arches in his sign, making a play on the real McDonald's. He was forced to remove the arches and add Norman in front of McDonald's on the sign so as not to appear affiliated with the chain.

Q34   In which one of the following circumstance, is McDonald's most likely to win a 'passing off' lawsuit?

A.   A breach of copyright law in using the term Mc.
B.   Having the surname McDonald's as part of a sign's name.
C.   Using McDonald's established reputation to benefit trade.
D.   Any type of business placing Mc in front of its name.

Answer [   ]

Q35 In 2004, McDonald's filed a lawsuit against the fast-food restaurant McJoy in the Philippines. Which of the following was the most likely outcome of the court's decision?

A. McJoy changed its name to MyJoy.
B. McJoy retained its name.
C. McJoy was fined for defamation of the McDonald's name.
D. McDonald's lost the case and had to pay the court costs.

Answer

Section 2 Scientific knowledge and applications

Mock test 2

27 questions
Time allowed 30 minutes
No calculators

In this mock test, all of the questions come with their revision topics shown in parentheses. For example, (P3b; M6d) means revise Physics topic 3b and Maths topic 6d; (B1a; C10b,c) means revise Biology topic 1a and Chemistry topics 10b and 10c. Some questions include a hint indicating the method of solution.

Q1   (B1b; B5a) Below are three statements about the pancreas:

i)   Insulin is produced in the pancreas in the islets of Langerhans, and is a hormone.

ii)   Amylase is also produced in the salivary glands.

iii)   The majority of digestive enzymes are secreted by the pancreas.

Creon is a medication used to treat sufferers of pancreatitis, which results in the reduction of substances produced in the pancreas. Assuming that Creon is medication which can only be taken orally, what effective substances are contained within Creon?

A.   Lipase, protease.
B.   Lipase, protease, insulin
C.   Lipase, protease, amylase
D.   Amylase, Lipase, Insulin
E.   Protease, Lipase, Insulin

Answer [   ]

Q2   (P6d or P8d) A golf ball is hit from a tee. The vertical component of its velocity is 30 metres per second (m s^{-1}). Calculate the maximum height that it will reach, ignoring the influence of spin and air resistance. (1 kg = 10 N.)

(hint: energy)

Answer [   ]

Q3   (B3) Look at the list (1 to 7) below and then choose the correct path for blood flowing through the heart to the lungs.

1. right ventricle; 2. bicuspid valve (mitral); 3. right atrium; 4. pulmonary artery; 5. pulmonary vein; 6. left atrium; 7. tricuspid valve.

A.   1, 2, 3, 4
B.   6, 2, 1, 5
C.   3, 2, 1, 5
D.   3, 7, 1, 4
E.   3, 2, 1, 4

(hint: 'tricycle before bicycle')

Answer ⬚

Q4   (C4b) 95 RON unleaded petrol contains 95 per cent octane, which combusts to produce carbon dioxide and water according to the following equation:

$$2C_8H_{18} + aO_2 = bCO_2 + cH_2O.$$

How many moles of water are produced from one mole of octane?

(hint: b first)

Answer ⬚

Q5   (P12a,c) The head pivots on the atlas vertebra ('C1') at the top of the spine. The weight of the head acts 4 cm in front of the pivot and the neck muscles act 6 cm behind the pivot to support the weight. What is the force in newtons, to the nearest newton, exerted by the neck muscles to support a head weighing 4 kg? (Take $g = 10$ m s^{-2}.)

A.   6 N
B.   36 N
C.   60 N
D.   40 N
E.   27 N

(hint: balance)

Answer ⬚

Q6   (P4a) A motorist travels from Birmingham to Blackpool, a distance of 120 miles, at an average speed of 60 miles per hour and then leaves Blackpool and returns to Birmingham at an average speed of 40 miles per hour. What was the average speed for the round trip?

A.   45 mph.
B.   48 mph.
C.   50 mph.
D.   54 mph.
E.   58 mph.

(hint: time)

Answer

Q7   (C3a) Which one of the following elements will not form an ionic compound with fluorine?

A.   Potassium.
B.   Aluminium.
C.   Carbon.
D.   Caesium.

Answer

Q8   (P17d) What is the approximate cost of boiling 1.75 litres of water in a kettle that draws 13 amps at 230 volts for four minutes, if electricity costs 15 pence per kilowatt-hour?

A.   1 p
B.   0.5 p
C.   2 p
D.   3 p
E.   4 p

(hint: volume irrelevant)

Answer

Q9   (B2) Which of the following sequences describes one half of a complete cycle of breathing?

   A. Chest muscles contract, chest expands, chest pressure rises, air is expired.

   B. Chest muscles contract, chest contracts, chest pressure rises, air is expired.

   C. Chest muscles contract, chest expands, chest pressure falls, air is inspired.

   D. Chest muscles relax, chest contracts, chest pressure falls, air is expired.

   E. Chest muscles relax, chest expands, chest pressure falls, air is inspired.

Answer [   ]

Q10 (C1, 2) Choose the correct word or term (labelled A to K) from the list below to match each numbered space (i to vi) in the following text. Some words or terms may be used more than once or not at all.

A = element; B = mixture; C = molecules; D = ions; E = proton; F = atoms; G = charge; H = reduced; I = solution; J = compound; K = oxidized.

Sulphuric acid, H_2SO_4, is a [...i...] of hydrogen, oxygen and sulphur [...ii...]. It is manufactured by burning the [...iii...] sulphur in air to form [...iv...] of sulphur dioxide. These are then [...v...] to sulphur trioxide, which is absorbed in sulphuric acid to form oleum. Sulphuric acid dissociates (ionizes) fully in water, making it a powerful [...vi...] donor and an oxidizing agent.

i   = ...

ii = ...

iii = ...

iv = ...

v   = ...

vi = ...

Q11   (P13e,f) Mains water flows through a series of pipes and taps as shown below:

Choose the correct answer from the choices given.

A.   The water pressures at taps A, B and C are all equal.
B.   The water pressure at tap A is greater than at tap B.
C.   The water pressures at taps A and B are equal.
D.   The water pressure at tap A is less than at tap C.

(hint: incompressible; inverse law)

Answer

Q12   (M2c, M10) If $x = (y +1)^{0.25} + 0.5$, calculate the value of y when $x = 2.5$.

Answer

Q13   (B6) A schematic diagram of a nephron is shown below. Where is the concentration of salt the highest?

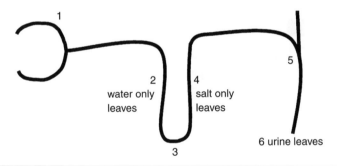

A.   1
B.   2
C.   3
D.   4
E.   5

Answer

Q14 (C6b) Which two of the following gases dissolve in water and turn litmus paper red?

A. O_2; B. CO; C. CO_2; D. HF; E. NH_3; F. CH_4.

Answer

Q15 (P18c,d, 17d) What is the total equivalent resistance for the resistors arranged below?

(hint: triple + pair + single)

Answer

Q16 (B8) According to the pedigree chart shown below, what is the probability of male M passing on an affected gene if he marries and has children, assuming that his wife is neither affected nor a carrier?

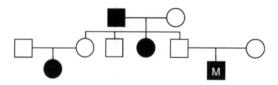

A.   100%.
B.   50%.
C.   33.3%.
D.   25%.
E.   0%.

Answer

Q17 (C5ii,iv) In a vehicle catalytic exhaust system the following pollutants are converted to less harmful emissions as follows:

i)   Carbon monoxide to carbon dioxide.
ii) Hydrocarbons to carbon dioxide and water.
iii) Nitrogen oxides to nitrogen and oxygen.

Select the correct option (A to F) from the table below to describe the chemical reactions taking place in i), ii) and iii).

	Chemical reaction		
	i	ii	iii
A	oxidation	reduction	reduction
B	oxidation	de-hydration	reduction
C	reduction	oxidation	reduction
D	oxidation	oxidation	reduction
E	oxidation	reduction	oxidation

Answer [   ]

Q18 (P7b) The three-car train shown below accelerates at 0.4 m s⁻². What is the tension in each of the three couplings?

0.4 m s⁻² →

| 10 tonnes | iii | 15 tonnes | ii | 20 tonnes | i |

A. i) 8 kN   ii) 6 kN   iii) 4 kN
B. i) 18 kN   ii) 18 kN   iii) 18 kN
C. i) 18 kN   ii) 12 kN   iii) 8 kN
D. i) 18 kN   ii) 10 kN   iii) 4 kN

(hint: independently for each coupling)

Answer [   ]

Q19 (M10, 11) A wallet contains £400 in £5, £10 and £20 notes. The number of £10 notes is twice the number of £5 notes and there are six fewer £20 notes than £10 notes. How many £5 notes are there?

Answer

Q20 (C10b,c) Which *two* of the following statements are true about propene?

A. It is an alkane.
B. It burns in air to produce carbon monoxide and hydrogen.
C. It is an unsaturated hydrocarbon.
D. It has carbon–carbon triple bonds.
E. It turns bromine water colourless.

Answer

Q21 (B2) The oxygen dissociation curve shows the percent saturation of haemoglobin versus the oxygen partial pressure. Which *two* of the following statements are true if the curve shifts to the right (dotted line) when a person begins to exercise?

A. There is an increase in the oxygen saturation of haemoglobin at the lungs.
B. There is a decrease in the oxygen saturation of haemoglobin at the tissues.
C. There is an increase in the partial pressure of oxygen at the tissues.
D. There is a decrease in the oxygen saturation of haemoglobin at the lungs.
E. There is a decrease in the partial pressure of oxygen at the tissues.

(hint: for tissues compare 50% Hb saturation values; for lungs compare $P_{50\%}$ values)

Answer

Q22 (M18b) Which of the following values of x satisfy the inequality $x(x - 3) \leq 10$?

    A. −3, −2, −1, 1, 0, 1, 2
    B. 1, 2, 3, 4, 5, 6, 7
    C. −4, −3, −2, −1, 0, 1
    D. −1, 0, 1, 2, 3, 4, 5
    E. 5, 6, 7, 8, 9, 10

Answer

Q23 (C9) The apparatus below shows the electrolysis of sodium chloride solution using carbon (inert) electrodes. Choose the correct substance or equation (labelled A to F) from the list below to match each label on the diagram (i to iv).

A: $2OH^- = O_2 + 2H_2O + 4e^-$
B: $2H_2O + 4e^- = 4OH^- + H_2$
C: $2Cl^- = Cl_2 + 2e^-$
D: Na
E: Cl_2
F: H_2

i   =......
ii =......
iii =......
iv =......

Answer

Q24   (B7) How many strands of DNA are there in the chromosome shown below?

A.   0
B.   1
C.   2
D.   4
E.   8

Answer [   ]

Q25   (P16b) The energy of x-ray photons is given by $E = Fh$ where f is the frequency of the photons in hertz (Hz), h is Planck's constant (6.63×10^{-34}). If an x-ray photon has 1.2×10^{-15} joules of energy, how many photons are produced every second?

A. 1.8×10^{18}
B. 5.5×10^{48}
C. 4.0×10^{34}
D. 8.3×10^{20}
E. 2.5×10^{18}

(hint: Hz = s^{-1})

Answer [   ]

Q26   (M3, 4) Calculate $\dfrac{25 + \dfrac{1}{8}}{7 - \dfrac{3}{10}}$.

Answer [   ]

Q27   (C9b, P15) The specific heat capacity of a substance is the energy required to raise 1 g by 1 °C; for water it is 4.2 J g^{-1} °C^{-1}. The heat of vaporization of a substance is the energy required to convert 1 g of liquid at its boiling point to gas at the same temperature; for water it is 2.3 kJ g^{-1}. Calculate the amount of energy required to raise 1 kg of water at 0 °C to boiling point and convert 200 g of it to steam. Give your answer in kilojoules.

Answer [   ]

Section 3 Writing task

Mock test 3

Choose one question
Time allowed 30 minutes; you have one side of A4 paper.
No dictionaries

1. Modern medicine has far more to do with science than with art

What do you understand by the above statement? Develop a unified argument that contradicts this opinion. Can you reconcile medicine as both art and science?

2. A little knowledge is a dangerous thing (Alexander Pope)

What is the author implying by this statement? Can a lot of knowledge be a more dangerous thing? Write a unified essay that argues the value in having a little knowledge.

3. Few people are capable of expressing with equanimity opinions that differ from the prejudices of their social environment. Most people are even incapable of forming such opinions (Albert Einstein)

What does the author mean by these comments and how would you refute them? Write a unified essay that includes examples of prejudices and how changes in attitudes and beliefs can be brought about.

4. Having knowledge of an unethical act and allowing it to continue can spread an unwanted contagion to society (Bertrand Russell)

What contagion is the author referring to in this statement? Discuss the implications of the quote, using examples to illustrate supportive and refuting positions.

Section 1 Aptitude and skills

Mock test 4

35 questions
Time allowed one hour
No calculators

Q1   (A2, 3) Studies on longevity have found that children born to mothers aged 25 and below are likely to live the longest. Longevity is further increased if the child is the firstborn. Younger mums bear offspring that are healthier, thrive better and are less prone to infections.

Which one of the following might be inferred from the above paragraph?

A.   The ova of younger women are likely to be healthier than the ova of older women.
B.   Longevity is inversely proportional to the age of the mother.
C.   Mothers aged 25 and below are healthier than older mothers.
D.   Younger mothers bear a higher proportion of females than older mothers and females live longer.

Answer   [   ]

Q2   (A2, 3) We should all buy locally farmed produce to reduce carbon emissions. Flying food halfway around the world might benefit poor farmers in developing countries but it increases its carbon footprint.

Which of the following is an implicit assumption of the above argument?

A.   Food from poor farmers is flown halfway around the world.
B.   Locally produced food has the lower carbon footprint.
C.   Poor farmers are not as important as carbon emissions.
D.   Local farmers are more important than poor farmers.
E.   Buying local produce supports local farmers.

Answer   [   ]

Q3 (A2, 3) The answer to road congestion is not to build more roads. Road building has continued apace over the last 10 years but so has congestion because
the new roads have encouraged drivers to travel longer distances and make
more journeys.

Which one of the following, if true, would seriously weaken the above argument?

A. The money spent on public transport has declined over the last decade.
B. When more roads are built the traffic soon fills to the new capacity.
C. There are 5 million more vehicles on the road than there were a decade
    ago.
D. Economic activity has increased over the last 10 years.

Answer

Q4 (P5) The graph shows the motion of a car over seven time intervals H, I, J, K,
L and M.

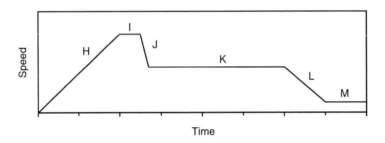

Which two intervals correspond with the greatest acceleration and the least
displacement (distance)?

A. H and I.
B. H and K.
C. J and I.
D. J and M.
E. H and M.

(hint: slopes and areas)

Answer

Q5   (M7b) A microwave oven is on sale with a 20 per cent discount. The following month the price is reduced by a further 10 per cent. What is the overall price reduction in percentage terms?

Answer _____

Q6   (A2, 3) More than 50 per cent of the prison population re-offend once they are released. Building more prisons and handing down longer sentences will significantly reduce crime.

Statement: 10 per cent of crimes reach court.

Which of the following best describes how the short statement relates to the argument?

A.   It lends significant support to the argument.
B.   It restates the conclusion of the argument.
C.   It restates one of the premises of the argument.
D.   It neither supports nor challenges the argument.
E.   It presents a significant challenge to the argument.

Answer _____

Q7   (A2, 3) The misuse of antibiotics has led to the spread of superbugs like MRSA. Doctors should know that most ear, nose and throat infections are self-limiting, which means that 90 per cent of prescriptions are unnecessary. The rise of superbugs is due to the over-eagerness of doctors to prescribe antibiotics.

Which one of the following shows that the conclusion is unsafe even if the evidence is correct?

A.   Patients with an infection expect their doctor to prescribe them antibiotics.
B.   In healthy people most MRSA infections are self-limiting.
C.   Doctors are only happy about writing prescriptions for the 10 per cent of patients who really need them.
D.   Superbugs would not have proliferated if antibiotics had not been over-prescribed.
E.   90 per cent of infections would have cleared up without the use of antibiotics.

Answer _____

Questions 8 to 9 refer to the following information:

Fruit juice has often been marketed as a health product, and it is easy to understand why. Fruit, from which juice is derived, is a relatively healthy balance of fibre, vitamins, minerals and sugars. In particular, the presence of fibre adds bulk, and slows the progression of digestion. This means that the sugars are absorbed over a prolonged period. Juice, on the other hand, misses out this key ingredient, but still contains the high sugar load. The issue here arises from the way our body reacts to sugar: if it detects too much, too fast, it releases a burst of insulin, a hormone which drives the sugar into muscles and converts them to stored energy. As you can imagine, juice is digested quickly, and the sugar stored as a result of the insulin. The result? Rapid weight gain and all of its consequences, from diabetes to cardiovascular risk. Fruit juice is not a health product, and should be avoided by most of the population.

Q8   Which of the following, if true, would strengthen the above argument?

A.   Fruit juice can be sold 'with pulp' which contains some fibre to slow digestion.

B.   Similar foods containing rapidly-absorbed sugars such as chocolate also cause weight gain.

C.   The cost of fruit juice prohibits most of the population from consuming it regularly.

D.   The manufacturing of concentrated fruit juice often adds sugar, whereas freshly pressed juice has no added sugar.

E.   Fruit juice is used by some people to replace other sweet products such as chocolate or candy.

Answer [   ]

Q9   Which of the following are key supporting arguments of the above passage?

   i)   The speed of absorption of sugar plays an important role in insulin secretion.

   ii) Digestion speed of liquids is different to that of solids.

   iii) The benefit of vitamins and minerals is offset by the negative aspect of sugar in fruit juice.

   A.   1 only
   B.   2 only
   C.   3 only
   D.   1 and 2 only
   E.   2 and 3 only
   F.   1, 2 and 3

Answer   [   ]

Q10 (M13a,b) Which pie chart might display the same data as the bar chart?

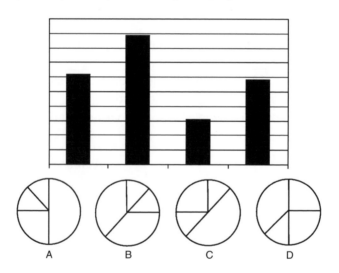

Answer   [   ]

Q11   (M13c) The line graph shows the trend in the number of households with regular use of a car from 1960 to 2000. The graph shows that the number of one-car-only households has been stable at 45 per cent from about 1970.

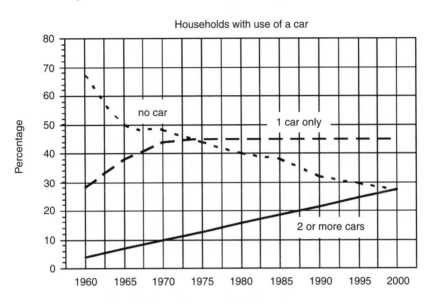

Households with use of a car

If trends continue, approximately when will the number of two or more car households equal the number of one-car households?

A. 2010
B. 2012
C. 2015
D. 2020
E. 2030

(hint: gradient)

Answer ☐

Q12   (M7b) By what fraction did no-car ownership decline between 1965 and 1995?

A. 1/5
B. 2/5
C. 1/2
D. 3/5
E. 4/5

Answer ☐

Q13 (M7b) If in the future, half of all households have the use of two or more cars, what percentage increase will this be compared with the 1970 figure?

    A. 40%.
    B. 400%.
    C. 450%.
    D. 500%.
    E. 550%.

Answer [   ]

Q14 (A2, 3) Common sense dictates that in the event of an accident, the driver of a smaller car is more likely to be injured than the driver of a large car. Therefore, it is preferable to drive a big, polluting car and ignore the damage to the environment than to drive a small, environmentally friendly car and put your own safety at risk.

Which of the following is an unwarranted assumption of the above argument?

    A. Car safety in an accident is a matter of common sense.
    B. Bigger cars usually burn more fuel than smaller cars.
    C. Personal safety is more important than damaging the environment.
    D. You should never put your own safety at risk.
    E. Occupants of smaller cars are more likely to be injured in an accident than occupants of larger cars.

Answer [   ]

Q15 (A2, 3) Discipline in schools has deteriorated since the abolishment of corporal punishment. School detention has not proved as effective as 'the cane' in deterring unruly behaviour. Disruptive pupils have a negative effect on the performance of a school because they reduce pupils' exposure to classroom instruction.

Which of the following can safely be inferred from the above paragraph?

    A. Rewarding desirable behaviour in the classroom will improve school performance.
    B. Poor performance in schools is linked with a lack of classroom discipline.
    C. Bringing back 'the cane' is the best way to improve pupil behaviour.
    D. Unruly behaviour is linked with anxiety over classroom performance.

Answer [   ]

Q16 (A2, 3) There is a clear link between MMR vaccinations and autism in children. The number of children diagnosed with autism has increased in proportion to the number of children receiving the triple vaccine. It can be concluded that an MMR vaccination increases the risk of a child developing autism.

Which of the following, if true, would show that the conclusion is unsafe even if the evidence is correct?

A.   It can be difficult to diagnose autism differentially from Asperger's syndrome.

B.   The number of cases of autism prior to the introduction of the MMR vaccine is unknown.

C.   The age when MMR is given coincides with the age when autism is first diagnosed.

D.   Many of the children diagnosed with autism have not had the MMR vaccine.

Answer [   ]

Q17 (A2, 3) Poverty in the UK can be defined in three ways: absolute, relative and social exclusion. People in absolute poverty are 'living below the breadline' with barely sufficient resources to sustain themselves. Relative poverty defines income and resources in relation to the national average (less than 60 per cent). Social exclusion is a new term that looks at the broader picture of unemployment, bad housing, crime levels, poor health and family breakdown as well as low incomes when attempting to define poverty.

Which of the following statements best summarizes the paragraph?

A.   No person in the UK is in absolute poverty, 60 per cent are in relative poverty and less than 40 per cent are socially excluded.

B.   Few people in the UK are in absolute poverty and those in relative poverty earn no more than 40 per cent of the national average wage.

C.   There are more people in relative poverty in the UK than there are in absolute poverty and social exclusion together.

D.   Poverty for the vast majority of people in the UK is a moral question concerned with the unequal distribution of resources in society.

E.   Poverty cannot be defined in terms of low incomes without including social factors.

Answer [   ]

Q18 (A2, 3) Improvements in teaching and investment in schools have led to an increase in the number of medical and veterinary school applicants achieving triple-A grades. As a result, universities now have to rely on selection tests as a means of differentiating between the most able candidates.

Which two of the following if true would most seriously weaken the above argument?

A. Exam boards have maintained exam standards at the same level for the past ten years.
B. Students do not have to work as hard as in the past.
C. Candidates sitting selection tests are achieving higher marks every year.
D. Exam boards are making A-levels easier to pass.
E. The exam marks of first-year university students are getting worse every year.

Answer _____

Q19 (M14a,b, M19c,i) The box and whisker plot summarizes the performance of 500 students in the first two sections of the BMAT.

3.4   3.9   5.1   6.9   8.7

What is the probability that if two students are chosen at random one will have achieved four marks or more and one will have achieved seven marks or more?

A. 1/2
B. 1/4
C. 1/8
D. 1/16
E. 3/16

Answer _____

Q20 (A2, 3) Place the following four sentences in the order in which they form the most coherent passage.

A. The need for bipedal locomotion may have arisen when climate change forced apes to live more on the ground than in the trees.
B. Another theory is that the brain grew after humans stopped walking on all fours.
C. Some anthropologists have hypothesized that the human brain developed when people began using their hands as tools.
D. Walking upright preceded development of the hand, which was then free to develop, unhindered by walking.

Answer [   ]

Q21 (M13b) The stacked bar chart shows the number of pupils with special educational needs (SEN) and without SEN in five schools, V, W, X, Y and Z.

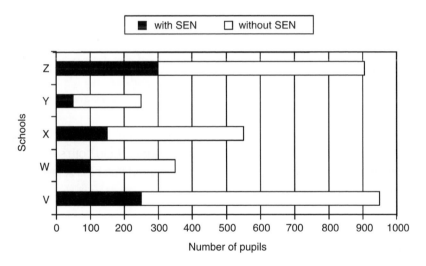

Which school had the lowest proportion of pupils without SEN?

A. Z
B. Y
C. X
D. W
E. V

Answer [   ]

Q22 (M13b) According to the stacked bar chart, what percent of the total pupils with SEN in all five schools are found among the *two* schools with the most pupils having SEN? Give your answer to the nearest whole percent.

A. 65%
B. 29%
C. 70%
D. 32%
E. 55%

Answer

Q23 (M13b, M7) If 40% of the pupils with SEN are on free school meals and there are a total of 426 pupils on free school meals in all five schools, what per cent of the pupils without SEN are *not* on free school meals?

A. 45%.
B. 12%.
C. 4%.
D. 8%.
E. 50%.

Answer

Q24 (A4a) Out of 18 candidates who sat a BMAT, 12 held an A level in Chemistry and 11 held an A level in Biology. Some candidates held both subjects and no candidate held neither subject. How many candidates held A-level Chemistry but not A-level Biology?

A. 4
B. 5
C. 6
D. 7
E. 8

(hint: two-circle problem; let n = the overlap)

Answer

Q25 (M10a,b) What volume of 1.0 molar saline solution must be added to 500 ml of 6.0 molar saline solution to dilute it to a 2.0 molar solution? (1 molar = 1 mol/L)

A. 750 ml
B. 1.0 L
C. 1.5 L
D. 1.75 L
E. 2.0 L

(hint: algebra; add x litres; moles constant)

Answer

Q26 (M13e) Anti-hypertensive drugs are an important method of controlling high blood pressure (BP). There are four main *classes* of drug, namely ACE inhibitors (A), beta-blocker (B), calcium channel blockers (C) and diuretics (D). Table 1 shows the preferred choice of drugs as well as those to avoid (contraindicated).

Table 2 shows which treatment options are preferred in patients with diabetes. ACE inhibitors (A) are the first choice of treatment and these can be combined with other classes of drugs to provide a sufficient reduction in blood pressure.

Table 1: Anti-hypertensive drugs: indications and contraindications

	Indicated in:	Contraindicated in:
class A	heart failure, CHD	renovascular disease, pregnancy
class B	angina, MI	asthma, COPD, heart block
class C	angina	heart block, heart failure
class D	heart failure	gout

legend: CHD = coronary heart disease; MI = myocardial infarction; COPD = chronic obstructive pulmonary disease

Table 2: Treatment options for BP control in patients with diabetes

	Treatment options
Step 1	A
Step 2	A + C
Step 3	A + C + D
Step 4	A + C + D + F

legend: A = ACE inhibitor; B = beta-blocker; C = calcium channel blocker; D = thiazide diuretic; F = furosemide diuretic

According to Tables 1 and 2, what would be the next treatment option for a patient with diabetes and heart failure, whose blood pressure remains elevated despite ACE inhibitor therapy?

A. Beta-blocker.
B. Calcium channel blocker.
C. Thiazide diuretic.
D. Calcium channel blocker + diuretic.
E. Furosemide diuretic.

Answer

Q27 A patient with diabetes, angina and asthma remains hypertensive despite ACE inhibitor therapy. What would be the next treatment option to consider?

A. Beta-blocker.
B. Calcium channel blocker.
C. Thiazide diuretic.
D. Calcium channel blocker + diuretic.
E. Furosemide diuretic.

Answer

Q28 In a darts tournament two teams of 16 players each are drawn against each other and the winners go forward to the next round. Two players fail to turn up and their opponents are given an automatic win. What is the total number of matches that will have to be played to find a winner?

A. 32
B. 31
C. 30
D. 29
E. 28

Answer

Q29 (M10a) A round of toast and a portion of margarine cost £1.10. The toast costs £1 more than the margarine. How much does the round of toast cost?

A. £0.90
B. £0.95
C. £1.00
D. £1.05
E. £1.15

Answer

Q30 (M9a,e) A solid sphere fits neatly inside a hollow cube. The volume of the sphere is given by its radius cubed multiplied by four-thirds pi (π). What is the ratio of the volume of the sphere to the volume of the cube?

A. 6π
B. $32/3\pi$
C. $2/3\pi$
D. $6/\pi$
E. $\pi/6$

Answer

Q31   (A2, 3) Tax on cigarettes means that smokers' contributions to the economy far outweigh what they cost the NHS in treating smoking-related diseases. Therefore, the tax raised on smoking benefits the economy for both smokers and non-smokers alike.

Which of the following, if true, identifies the most significant flaw in the argument's conclusion?

A.   Tax raised on cigarettes is not necessarily spent on the NHS.
B.   The money smokers would save by not smoking would generate other tax revenues for the economy.
C.   The social costs of smoking and the suffering it causes far outweigh the financial benefits.
D.   The money spent on smokers is not limited to NHS treatment.

Answer

Q32   (A2, 3) Patients cannot undergo medical treatment without first giving their informed consent, either implied, verbal or written. However, in a medical emergency when a patient is unconscious, consent to treatment may be presumed unless there has been a prior expression of a refusal to consent in that emergency situation.

If the paragraph is true, which of the following statements must be false?

A.   Patients must know what they are consenting to and have the right to refuse medical interventions.
B.   Consent is never presumed in a conscious patient but is normally presumed in an unconscious patient.
C.   The patient's prior wish to refuse treatment is often ignored in situations where there is a risk to the patient's life.
D.   Doctors are sometimes allowed to act in what they know to be the best interests of their patients.
E.   Doctors must always act to save the patient's life unless the patient has explicitly forbidden it in writing.

Answer

Q33 (P4a) Zak cycles to university at an average speed of 12 miles per hour and Phoebe walks the same route at an average speed of 3 miles per hour. If Phoebe sets out at 08.30 hrs and Zak sets out 15 minutes later, what time will it be when he catches her up?

   A. 08.45

   B. 08.50

   C. 08.55

   D. 09.00

   E. 09.05

(hint: same distance d; Phoebe: $d = st$; Zak $d = ?$)

Answer [   ]

Questions 34 and 35 refer to the following information:

People who abuse alcohol are motivated to reduce their consumption when the adverse consequences outweigh the perceived benefits. Disulfiram (Antabuse®) is an adjunct therapy that is used to help maintain abstinence in patients who abuse alcohol. People who consume even a small amount of alcohol after taking disulfiram medication experience symptoms similar to a 'hangover', including nausea and vomiting, which makes the drug a powerful alcohol deterrent; a 12-hour period of abstinence is necessary before commencing disulfiram therapy. Alcoholism is a disease characterized by dependency where the abuser is no longer able to control his/her intake and cannot stop drinking under any circumstances.

Research suggests that genetics and a family history of alcoholism predispose some people to dependency; other people remain free of dependency. Alcohol-induced liver disease can progress from steatosis (fatty liver), to alcoholic hepatitis and finally alcoholic cirrhosis. Steatosis is reversible when the drinking stops. Drinking heavily for longer periods may give rise to alcoholic hepatitis where fat becomes inflamed and the damage takes several weeks to resolve after the patient stops drinking. In alcoholic cirrhosis the damaged cells are replaced by permanent scar tissue and if the drinking continues, the consequences can be fatal.

Patients with alcoholic liver disease may present with jaundice, hepatic encephalopathy (damage to the brain and nervous system) and ascites (fluid in the abdomen), which is caused by portal vein hypertension. The blood pressure increases in the portal vein because the blood cannot flow normally from the digestive organs to the liver. Portal vein hypertension may lead to oesophageal varices (dilated veins), and if these rupture, the mortality rate is very high.

Q34   Which two of the following statements can be inferred from the passage?

   A.   Disulfiram is not the primary treatment for alcohol abuse.
   B.   Disulfiram is unsuitable for patients who are dependent on alcohol.
   C.   Alcoholism can run in families though there is no genetic trait.
   D.   Any alcohol-induced liver disease is reversible if the patient stops in time.

   Answer [   ]

Q35   Which two of the following statements can be inferred from the passage?

   A.   Chronic alcohol abuse eventually leads to dependency.
   B.   Chronic alcohol abuse may lead to brain damage.
   C.   Alcohol abuse is a disease process.
   D.   The hepatic portal vein drains blood from the liver.
   E.   A swollen abdomen and a jaundiced appearance are consistent with alcohol abuse or alcohol dependency.

   Answer [   ]

Section 2 Scientific knowledge and applications

Mock test 5

27 questions
Time allowed 30 minutes
No calculators

Q1 Below are three statements relating to female sex hormones and the menstrual cycle:

i) A hormone produced by the corpus luteum inhibits production of Leuteinising Hormone (LH).

ii) The secretion of oestrogen, a hormone produced by the ovaries, is stimulated by Follicle Stimulating Hormone (FSH).

iii) A hormone produced by the corpus luteum inhibits production of Follicle Stimulating Hormone (FSH).

Which of the following statements regarding the human menstrual cycle are correct?

A. i only
B. ii only
C. iii only
D. i and ii only
E. i and iii only
F. All three

Answer _____

Q2   (P20b) A radioisotope is being used for a medical procedure. The table shows how the sample decays with time. What was the activity of the sample when it was prepared?

Time: days	Activity: counts per minute
0	
1	3.2×10^5
2	8×10^4
3	2×10^4
4	5000

A. 6.4×10^4
B. 1.28×10^6
C. 2.56×10^6
D. 5.12×10^5

(hint: half-life)

Answer [   ]

Q3   (B3) Identify the correct path for blood flowing through the heart to the body.

A. Left atrium, tricuspid valve, left ventricle, aorta.
B. Left atrium, bicuspid (mitral) valve, left ventricle, pulmonary artery.
C. Left atrium, bicuspid (mitral) valve, left ventricle, aorta.
D. Right atrium, pulmonary valve, right ventricle, pulmonary artery.
E. Right atrium, tricuspid valve, right ventricle, pulmonary artery.

Answer [   ]

Q4   (C5ii) In which of the following compounds does oxygen have the highest oxidation number?

A. H_2O
B. O_2
C. H_2O_2
D. CO_2
E. OF_2

(hint: 0, –, +)

Answer [   ]

Q5   (P10a,7e) A golf ball of mass 46 g is hit from a tee peg at a speed of 50 m s^{-1}. If the ball is in contact with the golf club for 10 milliseconds, what force is exerted on the club face?

(hint: change in momentum)

Answer [   ]

Q6   (M9a) If the area of the square is 9 cm^2, what is the area of the circle?

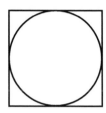

A. 2π
B. 2.25π
C. 2.5π
D. 3π
E. 3.25π

Answer [   ]

Q7   (C1, 2) Which of the following statements could be true for the element krypton?

A.   36 protons, 36 neutrons, 36 electrons, 6 isotopes.
B.   83.8 protons and neutrons and 36 electrons.
C.   36 protons and 36 electrons, 6 isotopes.
D.   6 isotopes, 36 protons, 36 electrons, 84 neutrons.

Answer [   ]

Q8 (P18d) In the diagram, what current flows through the bulb?

A. 1 A
B. 4 A
C. 3 A
D. 8 A
E. 6 A

(hint: parallel; bulb)

Answer

Q9 (B5) Choose the correct word or term (labelled A to K) from the list below to match each numbered space (i to ix) in the following text. Some words may be used more than once or not at all.

A = pituitary; B = less; C = metabolism; D = more; E = hypothalamus; F = hot; G = endocrine; H = hormones; I = cold; J = thyroid; K = exocrine

The [...i...] is the gland of the [...ii...] system responsible for [...iii...]. It secretes the [...iv...] T3 and T4 into the bloodstream in response to thyroid-stimulating hormone (TSH) released by the [...v...] gland. This latter gland is adjacent to and regulated by the [...vi...] region of the brain. Thus in [...vii...] weather the brain signals the [...viii...] gland to release [...ix...] TSH.

i   = ...
ii   = ...
iii = ...
iv   = ...
v   = ...
vi   = ...
vii = ...
viii = ...
ix   = ...

Q10 (C10b) Bromine water can be used to distinguish between alkanes and alkenes because bromine reacts with alkenes by adding to both sides of the double bond. Which two of the following hydrocarbons will turn bromine water colourless?

    A. C_2H_6
    B. C_3H_6
    C. $C_{12}H_{26}$
    D. $C_{20}H_{42}$
    E. $C_{60}H_{120}$

(hint: draw/general formula?)

Answer ▭

Q11 (P8a,b) Ali (A), Ben (B), Chris (C) and Dave (D) lift weights at the gym.
Ali can lift 25 kg 12 times in 20 seconds.
Ben can lift 35 kg 10 times in 35 seconds.
Chris can lift 40 kg 5 times in 20 seconds.
Dave can lift 60 kg once in 5 seconds.

Choose the correct answer A, B, C or D if all the weights are lifted through a distance of 1 metre.

(hint: work done)

    A. Dave uses the least energy but develops the most power.
    B. Ben uses the most energy and develops the most power.
    C. Ali develops the most power but does not use the most energy.
    D. Chris uses more energy than Dave and develops more power than him.

Answer ▭

Q12 (M6) What is $5.2 \times 10^{12} + 4.8 \times 10^{11} - 1.0 \times 10^{10}$ in scientific notation?

    A. 5.68×10^{12}
    B. 5.67×10^{12}
    C. 5.67×10^{11}
    D. 56.7×10^{10}
    E. 5.60×10^{12}

Answer ▭

Q13 (P13a, 3e) Lead ingots measuring 200 mm × 100 mm × 50 mm are stacked with their largest face on the ground. (1 kg = 10 N.)

200 mm

100 mm

50 mm

If the density of lead is approximately 11 gram per cm³, what pressure in pascals (Pa) will an ingot exert on the ground?

(hint: 1 Pa = 1 N m⁻²)

Answer

Q14 (B6) A schematic diagram of a nephron is shown below. Identify the correct transport processes from 1 through to 5.

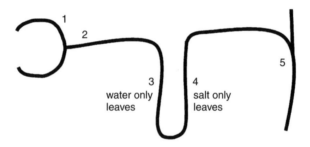

3
water only
leaves

4
salt only
leaves

A. Ultrafiltration, active transport, osmosis, active transport, osmosis.
B. Diffusion, active transport, osmosis, active transport, osmosis.
C. Ultrafiltration, re-absorption, countercurrent, active transport, excretion.
D. Ultrafiltration, osmosis, active transport, osmosis, diffusion.
E. Ultrafiltration, re-absorption, diffusion, active transport, active transport.

Answer

Q15 (C7iii) The pH of blood is maintained at 7.4 by the carbonic acid hydrogen carbonate ion buffer as follows:

$CO_2 + H_2O = H^+ + HCO_3^-$.

Which of the following statements is consistent with respiratory acidosis of the blood?

A. CO_2 levels rise and the pH falls.
B. CO_2 levels rise and the pH remains unchanged.
C. CO_2 levels rise and the pH rises.
D. CO_2 levels fall and the pH rises.

Answer ☐

Q16 (C9iii) The apparatus below shows the electrolysis of a strong solution of hydrochloric acid using carbon (inert) electrodes. Choose the correct substance or equation (labelled A to G) from the list below to match each label on the diagram (i to iv):

A: $2OH^- \rightarrow O_2 + 2H_2O + 4e^-$
B: $2H^+ + 2e^- \rightarrow H_2$
C: $2Cl^- \rightarrow Cl_2 + 2e^-$
D: Na
E: Cl_2
F: H_2
G: O_2

i   = ...
ii = ...
iii = ...
iv = ...

Q17   (B8) What type of inheritance is shown in the diagram below if F is not a carrier for the disease?

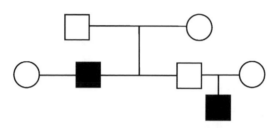

key: male = ☐ female = ◯ affected/disease = shaded

A.   Autosomal dominant.
B.   Autosomal recessive.
C.   X-linked dominant.
D.   X-linked recessive.
E.   Autosomal recessive or X-linked recessive.

Answer

Q18   (P7a,b,e) A rightward force is applied to a 12-kg object to move it across a rough surface at constant velocity. The object encounters 30 N of frictional force.

$(g = 10 \text{ m s}^{-2})$
Use the diagram to determine to the following forces:

A.   gravitational force = ...
B.   normal force = ...
C.   applied force = ...
D.   net force = ...

(hint: Newton's three laws: acceleration?)

Answer

Q19   (M9a) What is the area of the shaded region if the diameter of the circle is x?

A. $x^2 - \pi x^2$

B. $x^2(1 - 4\pi)$

C. $x^2(1 - \pi)/4$

D. $x^2(4 - \pi)/4$

E. $x^2 \pi /4 - \pi$

Answer _____

Q20   (C10c) Choose the word or term (labelled A to I) from the list below to match each numbered space (i to v) in the following text. Some words or terms may be used more than once or not at all.

A = melting points; B = boiling points; C = densities; D = volatile; E = hydrocarbon; F = inorganic; G = liquid; H = top; I = bottom.

Fractional distillation of crude oil relies on the difference in the [...i...] of the [...ii...] constituents. The more [...iii...] fractions have the lowest [...iv...] and go to the [...v...] of the tower.

i   = ...

ii = ...

iii = ...

iv = ...

v   = ...

Q21 (B4a,b) Which of the following sequences describes the path of a nerve impulse in a reflex arc?

A. Receptor, efferent neurone, PNS, motor neurone, effector.
B. Receptor, afferent neurone, PNS, motor neurone, effector.
C. Receptor, effector, CNS, afferent neurone, efferent neurone.
D. Receptor, efferent neurone, CNS, afferent neurone, effector.
E. Receptor, afferent neurone, CNS, efferent neurone, effector.

(hint: 'efferent' away (from brain))

Answer

Q22 (P7b,d) In a hammer-throwing contest a competitor whirls a mass of 4 kg around her body in a circle. If the speed of rotation of the hammer is one revolution per second before letting go, what is the size of the force acting on the competitor's arms? The acceleration (a) of a rotating mass (m) towards the centre of rotation is given by $a = v^2/r$ where r is the radius of the circle and v the tangential velocity.

A. $16\pi^2 r$ N
B. $8\pi^2 r$ N
C. $4\pi r$ N
D. πr N
E. $8\pi^2 r^2$ N

(hint: speed, distance, time)

Answer

Q23 (M19, 20) Five cards are picked in turn from a shuffled pack of 52 playing cards. The first four cards are the Jack of Spades, King of Hearts, Queen of Diamonds and Jack of Clubs. What is the probability that the next card will not be another face (court) card?

A. 1/6
B. 5/6
C. 12/52 × 11/51 × 10/50 × 9/49
D. 5/52
E. 1/13

Answer

Q24 (B8(1)) Choose the word or term (labelled A to I) from the list below to match each numbered space (i to vi) in the following text. Some words or terms may be used more than once or not at all.

A = gene; B = genotype; C = chromosome; D = homozygous; E = allele; F = heterozygous; G = phenotype; H = zygote.

In determining inheritance, a [...i...] is a section of a [...ii...] that codes for a particular protein or characteristic. Each [...iii...], dominant or recessive, determines the type of coding for a trait. If these are the same the [...iv...] will have a homozygous [...v...] but if they are different the dominant one will determine the [...vi...].

i =.......

ii =.......

iii =.......

iv =.......

v =.......

vi =.......

Q25 (C2) Nitric oxide reacts with oxygen to produce nitrogen dioxide according to the following equation:

$2NO_{(g)} + O_{2(g)} = 2NO_{2(g)}$

Which one of the following statements is false?

A. Nitric oxide is a mixture of nitrogen and oxygen.
B. Oxygen is an element and a diatomic molecule.
C. Nitrogen dioxide is a compound and a molecule.
D. The mass of reactants equals the mass of products.
E. Three moles of reactants produce two moles of products.

Answer _____

Q26   What is the length of the diagonal line drawn inside the cube of side x?

A. $2x$
B. $x\sqrt{2}$
C. $x\sqrt{3}$
D. $3\sqrt{2}x$
E. $(x/2)\sqrt{3}$

(hint: extra line; Pythag. two triangles)

Answer ⬚

Q27   (C9, P14a, P15) The graph shows the time–temperature curve of pure water when heated at atmospheric pressure.

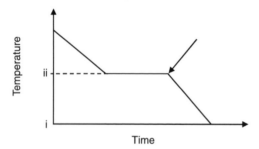

Which of the following statements are true and which are false?

A.   There is one phase with two phase changes.
B.   The temperature at i must be 273 K.
C.   The temperature at ii must be 373 K.
D.   Adding impurities to the water will increase ii.
E.   The temperature at ii is lower on Mount Everest.

A.   ......
B.   ......
C.   ......
D.   ......
E.   ......

Section 3 Writing task

Mock test 6

Choose one question
Time allowed 30 minutes; you have one side of A4 paper
No dictionaries

1. If we knew what we were doing, it would not be called research, would it? (Albert Einstein)

What do you think the author means by this? Can you advance a counter-argument? Are new facts derived from experimental research or are they derived from what is already known?

2. The female of the species is no longer the weaker sex

Explain what you believe the author means in making this statement. Discuss the claim in relation to men and women. Provide examples that support or refute the statement.

3. Medicine is a science of uncertainty and an art of probability (William Osler)

What does the author mean by this statement? How might his view relate to diagnosis and decision making?

4. What one generation finds ridiculous, the next accepts; and the third shudders when it looks back on what the first did (Peter Singer)

What is the author suggesting? Can you give examples of when this is truthful? Are there times when this is not applicable?

Section 1 Aptitude and skills

Mock test 7

35 questions
Time allowed one hour
No calculators

Q1 (P5) The graph shows the motion of a power-boat over six time intervals H, I, J, K, L and M.

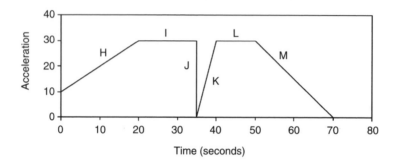

In which time interval is the change in velocity of the power-boat the greatest?

A. H
B. I
C. J
D. K
E. L
F. M

Answer [   ]

Q2 (M7b) A jeweller buys a watch and marks the price up 80 per cent before selling it to a customer. What percentage of the customer's price is the jeweller's purchase cost? Give your answer to the nearest whole number.

Answer [   ]

Q3   (A2, 3) Fractures of the hip are a leading cause of disability and mortality in elderly people. A high proportion of these patients have osteoporosis, which leads to fragile bones. All elderly people should take calcium and vitamin D supplements to help to prevent osteoporosis. This inexpensive treatment will reduce the risk of a hip fracture after a fall.

Which one of the following, if true, would seriously weaken the above argument?

A.   Most falls in the elderly do not lead to bone fractures.
B.   Preventive treatments are not cost-effective.
C.   Most fractures involve vertebrae and not the hip.
D.   Most elderly people do not have falls.
E.   Regular exercise is the best way to strengthen bones.

Answer [   ]

Q4   (A2, 3) Placebo-controlled drug trials are unethical if participants are denied new therapeutic treatments that might prove effective. Any new treatment should be tested alongside the existing standard therapies to offer candidates the possibility of a better outcome and not just a 'nothing' treatment.

Which two of the following, if true, would most seriously weaken the above argument?

A.   There is no guarantee that any new treatment will be any more effective than a placebo.
B.   It is unethical to employ treatments that have not been proven safe or effective in a placebo-controlled drug trial.
C.   In a placebo-based drug trial the participant loses the benefit of the standard treatment.
D.   Placebo treatments are frequently effective and should not be described as 'nothing' treatments.

Answer [   ]

Q5   (A2, 3) A five-year study has shown that obesity is caused by a sedentary lifestyle and not by over-eating. Participants with sedentary lifestyles put on more weight than participants who ate more.

Which of the following statements, if true, would make the findings of the study unsafe?

A.   Participants who put on more weight also dieted more.
B.   Participants who over-ate preferred fast food.
C.   Not all of the participants with a sedentary lifestyle put on weight.
D.   A sedentary lifestyle led to an increased food intake.
E.   A few participants lost weight during the five-year study.

Answer

Q6   (M3a) If the shapes drawn below are placed inside the square frame, what fraction of the frame will be empty?

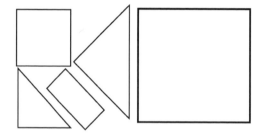

A.   1/16
B.   1/10
C.   1/8
D.   1/6
E.   1/4

Answer

Q7 Norton is west of Nettlestone, which is east of Niton. Ningwood is east of Norton and west of Niton. Newbridge is east of Niton, which is west of Norwood.

Norwood must be east of:

A. Norton, Ningwood and Niton.
B. Norton, Ningwood but not necessarily Niton.
C. Norton, Ningwood, Niton and Newbridge.
D. Ningwood, Niton and Newbridge only.
E. Norton, Ningwood and Niton but west of Newbridge.

(hint: horizontal line)

Answer [   ]

Q8 (M20) A 50-year-old woman has an abnormal mammogram. Use the probability tree to calculate the chances she has of having breast cancer (CB). Give your answer as a percentage to one decimal place.

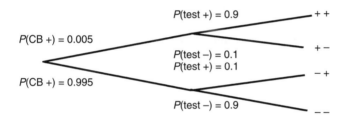

P(test +) = 0.9   + +

P(CB +) = 0.005

P(test −) = 0.1   + −
P(test +) = 0.1

− +
P(CB +) = 0.995

P(test −) = 0.9   − −

A. 4.3 per cent.
B. 4.4 per cent.
C. 4.5 per cent.
D. 4.8 per cent.
E. 5.0 per cent.

(hint: true positive + false positive; 1.0 = 100 per cent)

Answer [   ]

Q9   (M13b) The bar chart shows the proportion of excess winter deaths by age and sex in England and Wales.

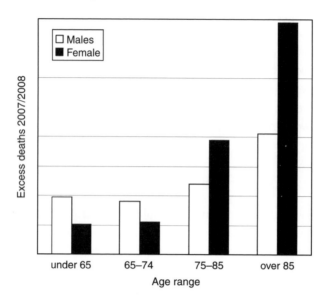

In percentage terms, approximately how many fewer male excess winter deaths were there than female excess winter deaths?

A.   26%.
B.   28%.
C.   32%.
D.   36%.
E.   40%.

Answer [   ]

Q10   (M13) Which of the columns in the table shows the correct number of excess winter deaths per 1000 of population consistent with the bar chart?

Age range	A	B	C	D	E
under 65	2	1	3	3	3
65–74	1.9	1.2	2.9	2.9	2.9
75–85	2.2	3.9	6.1	6.1	6.9
over 85	4.1	7.9	12	7.9	14

Answer [   ]

Q11 (M13) If there are approximately 25 000 excess deaths in total, how many of these were females aged 85 or over?

A. 6250
B. 8300
C. 10 000
D. 12 500
E. 15 000

Answer

Q12 (M7a) Estimate the population of England and Wales if the 25 000 excess deaths represent 0.048 per cent of the population.

A. 50 million.
B. 51 million.
C. 52 million.
D. 53 million.
E. 54 million.

Answer

Q13 (A2, 3) 'Grey power' is increasing at an alarming rate. More than a third of UK voters are now over age 55. Furthermore, the tendency for young people not to vote means that older people will constitute 50 per cent of the active voters by 2020. This might not matter if older voters acted in the best interests of society but they do not. Older people want increased pensions, better health-care and free public transport for the elderly, and it is the young who are going to have to pay for it.

Which of the following best summarizes the argument?

A. Older people are motivated by self-interest and expect young people to pay for their needs.
B. The increasing proportion of older people in society has made them a powerful interest group.
C. An increasingly older electorate will act in their own interests to ensure more resources are allocated to them.
D. Taxes will have to rise if the needs of older people are going to be met.

Answer

Q14 (A2, 3) Studies suggest that the more violence and aggression teenagers watch on television, the more aggressive they are likely to be to the people around them. Violent computer games also promote violence and these should be banned altogether. The best way to reduce real-life violence is to restrict teenagers' access to images of violence on the screen.

Which of the following is the best statement of the flaw in the above argument?

A. It would be better to modify children's attitudes towards violence and aggression before restricting access to it.

B. Children have the same human rights as adults and can choose what they want to watch on television.

C. Several childhood factors are known to influence teenage aggression.

D. Parents have a responsibility to moderate the viewing habits of their children.

E. Only children with prior psychiatric disorders are likely to exhibit aggressive tendencies.

Answer ⬚

Q15 (A2, 3) There has been a 10 per cent decline in the number of people taking out a gym membership. As a nation we are becoming less interested in fitness.

Which of the following is an implicit assumption of the above argument?

A. Ten per cent of people leaving gyms are not interested in fitness.

B. Gym membership is the best way of maintaining fitness.

C. Unless you work out at a gym you will not keep fit.

D. Ninety per cent of people join gyms to keep fit.

E. Unless you join a gym you are not interested in fitness.

Answer ⬚

Q16   (A2, 3) Prostate-specific antigen (PSA) levels are raised in men with prostate cancer. A study suggests that PSA levels get diluted in obese men because of their greater blood volume. Consequently it can be too late to treat obese men who have prostate cancer detected by a PSA test.

Statement: The total amount of PSA in obese men with prostate cancer is higher than it is in men of average weight with prostate with cancer.

Which of the following best describes how the statement relates to the study?

A.   It neither supports nor challenges the argument.
B.   It is inconsistent with the findings of the study.
C.   It restates the conclusion of the argument.
D.   It restates one of the premises of the argument.
E.   It is consistent with the finding of the study.

Answer ☐

Q17   (M2c) In DNA fingerprinting, the probability of one band matching is given by $p = 0.5$, or 1 in 2. The probability of two bands matching is given by $p = (0.5)^2$ or 1 in 4. If the population of the UK is approximately 60 million, how many bands need to be compared to be confident that one match will not happen by chance?

A.   30 bands.
B.   26 bands.
C.   20 bands.
D.   14 bands.
E.   10 bands.

(hint: $(1/2)^x = 1/2^x$)

Answer ☐

Q18 (M14b) The box and whisker plot summarizes the performance of 200 students in the first two sections of the BMAT.

2.9   3.8   5.2   6.4   8.8

Indicate all the false statements:

A. At least one student achieved 8.8 marks on the BMAT scale.
B. Half the students scored between 3.8 and 6.4 marks.
C. One-quarter of the pupils scored more than 3.8 marks.
D. The mean mark was 5.2.
E. The probability that two students chosen at random achieved more than 6.4 marks is 6.25 per cent.

A. = ...
B. = ...
C. = ...
D. = ...
E. = ...

Q19 (M13a) A high-calorie drink is available to patients in neutral, vanilla and chocolate flavours. The pie chart shows the popularity of the three flavours amongst patients.

Key:
NP = no preference expressed
DL = disliked all three

Which one of the following columns might represent preferences expressed?

Flavour	A	B	C	D	E
neutral	30	90	160	500	160
vanilla	60	120	320	300	80
chocolate	120	400	320	200	280

Answer [   ]

Q20 (M13b) The stacked bar chart shows retailers' annual book sales in four categories: children's (CH), adult non-fiction (AN), adult special (AS) and adult fiction (AF).

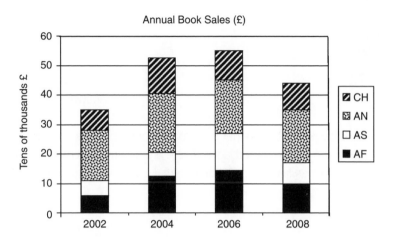

Annual Book Sales (£)

In which year did the smallest proportion of sales come from children's books?

A. 2002
B. 2004
C. 2006
D. 2008

Answer

Q21 (M7b) Approximately what is the increase in per cent in annual sales between the years with the greatest difference?

A. 20 per cent.
B. 40 per cent.
C. 49 per cent.
D. 57 per cent.
E. 66 per cent.

Answer

Q22 (M13b) According to the stacked bar chart, approximately what was the greatest increase in adult fiction sales over any two-year span?

A. £10 000
B. £60 000
C. £120 000
D. £150 000
E. £175 000

Answer [   ]

Q23 John has 36 books that are either paperbacks or hardbacks. One-quarter are fiction books and 24 are paperbacks. There are six times as many paperback non-fiction books as hardback fiction books. How many books does he have that are both hardback and non-fiction?

A. 2
B. 4
C. 6
D. 8
E. 9

(hint: 2 × 2 table; tally rows and columns)

Answer [   ]

Q24 (P3c) Water drips from a tap at a rate of one drop every three seconds. The volume of water in each drop is 0.1 ml. If the tap is left to drip for 25 hours, how many litres of water will be wasted?

Answer [   ]

Q25 Which shape does not belong with the other four?

A   B   C   D   E

Answer [   ]

Q26 (M2e,c) What is the missing number in the following series of numbers?
1, 2, 9, 64, 625, ?, 117 649.

A. 1110
B. 2048
C. 6072
D. 7776
E. 8824

Answer

Q27 (M13d) The scatter graph compares the BMAT test results of 25 candidates in Tests 1 and 2.

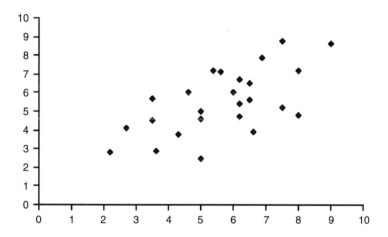

Which one of the following statements is true when comparing the test results in the two tests?

A. There is a strong positive correlation.
B. There is a weak negative correlation.
C. There is a weak positive correlation.
D. There is a strong negative correlation.
E. There is no correlation negative or positive.

Answer

Q28 (M3,4) If Paul can paint a house in six hours and Julie can paint a house in nine hours, how long will it take them to paint a house if they both work together?

A. 7 hours 30 minutes.
B. 4 hours 32 minutes.
C. 4 hours 24 minutes.
D. 3 hours 45 minutes.
E. 3 hours 36 minutes.

(hint: hourly rates)

Answer [   ]

Q29 (M2e) This is a code question. You have to break the code to work out the solution. If DICE = 3824 and DICE + FACE = 8848, then what number is represented by FACE – DACE?

A. 5026
B. 2000
C. 6824
D. 8500
E. 1400

Answer [   ]

Q30 (A2, 3) The hypothesis that the earth's atmosphere is warming because of anthropogenic greenhouse gases is clearly true. Carbon dioxide emitted from power stations and car exhausts is the principal culprit. Methane, the second most important greenhouse gas, arises from the decomposition of organic matter on agricultural farms.

Which one of the following, if true, would seriously weaken the above argument?

A. Climate change is a complex process and predicting it with any certainty is impossible in the short term.
B. Carbon dioxide makes up less than 0.05 per cent of the earth's atmosphere so it cannot be responsible for global warming.
C. Greenhouse gases released by human activities are not the primary source of greenhouse gases in the atmosphere.
D. A thousand years ago atmospheric temperatures were higher than today and anthropogenic greenhouse gases were lower.
E. Global warming did not begin until after the industrial revolution.

Answer [   ]

Questions 31 and 32 refer to the following passage:

Digoxin is a drug used by cardiologists to reduce the heart rate of patients. Why might you want to slow the heart rate down? This would be useful in cases of arrhythmia, abnormal and irregular rhythms which can put strain on the heart by making it beat too fast. The obvious downside of using a drug which slows the heart is that it might just slow it too much, causing heart failure and death.

Digoxin is a molecule of the same class as Digitalis, which importantly is the botanical name for the Foxglove from which that drug was derived. It is not clear how extracts from this plant first came to be used in a positive manner, but certainly it was used as a poison by early communities who discovered the potency of its fluid.

In recent times, patients who have been put on Digoxin by their doctors have run into some unusual issues. The problem comes when people take things which interact with digoxin in some way. The most classic example is that of grapefruit juice (often people living perfectly healthy lives will drink a glass each morning) and some were mysteriously found to be collapsed and dead on the floor.

This is because grapefruit, and those fruits in its family, contains an active substance, which acts on the liver to inhibit the P450 cytochrome enzyme system in the liver, which clears Digoxin in healthy patients. Drinking a glass of grapefruit juice per day allows Digoxin to build up to potentially dangerous levels, and slow the heart beyond the ability to sustain life. This problem has been so dangerous that Digoxin now comes with a warning against using it with grapefruit juice.

Pomegranate juice is in the same family, but is much less frequently consumed by people due to its high price. However, the increasing popularity of other positive benefits of pomegranate juice such as high levels of anti-oxidants means that it has become an increasingly popular beverage of choice.

Q31   Based on the above information, which of the following must be true about Digoxin?

i)   Digoxin is a plant-derived medication.
ii)   It has the same molecular weight as digitalis.
iii) It has been used therapeutically for considerable time.

A.   i only
B.   ii only
C.   iii only
D.   i and ii only
E.   i and iii only
F.   None of the above

Answer [   ]

Q32 Based on the information in the above passage alone, which of the following must be true?

    A. Because pomegranate juice is less frequently consumed, it poses less danger to individuals taking Digoxin than grapefruit juice.

    B. Pomegranate juice may not interact with cytochrome P450.

    C. High levels of antioxidants and other health benefits offset any risk of Digoxin interaction.

    D. Drinking pomegranate juice may result in sudden death in Digoxin takers.

    E. The price of pomegranate juice must be coming down.

                                                    Answer [   ]

Q33 (A2, 3) Chronic diseases are prevalent in the elderly population and 60 per cent of people attending GP surgeries with a chronic disease are aged 75 or above.

Which of the following is an implicit assumption of the above argument?

    A. Sixty per cent of elderly people attend their GP.

    B. Most elderly people attend their GP.

    C. The over-75s attend the GP the most frequently.

    D. Sixty per cent of elderly people have a chronic disease.

    E. Few people attending their GP are under 75.

                                                    Answer [   ]

Q34 (A2, 3) Sodium fluoride should not be added to drinking water as it is poisonous at trace levels, especially for children. Toothpastes and mouthwashes contain the warnings 'do not swallow' and 'children should be supervised' as evidence of this. Whilst sodium fluoride was an inexpensive method of preventing dental caries in the past, better dietary habits, oral hygiene and the presence of fluoride in toothpastes now make the fluoridation of drinking water unnecessary.

Which one of the following, if true, would seriously weaken the above argument?

A.   Some people cannot afford to buy toothpastes or fail to brush their teeth regularly.

B.   There are no reports of fluoridated water having harmed a child.

C.   The concentration of fluoride in drinking water is strictly controlled to be within safe limits.

D.   The benefits in preventing dental caries are only small.

E.   The safe limit for fluoride ion concentration is an arbitrary figure.

Answer [   ]

Q35   (A2, 3) Place the following four sentences in the order in which they form the most coherent passage.

A.   This produces a metal that is harder, more durable and easier to cast than copper.

B.   Thus, the earliest classification system for tool making refers to a Stone Age, a Bronze Age and an Iron Age, with the very brief Copper Age omitted.

C.   The Bronze Age ended when metallurgists found how to extract iron from its ore and forge it.

D.   When humans first started making metal tools they used copper, followed soon afterwards by bronze, which is copper alloyed with tin.

Answer [   ]

Section 2 Scientific knowledge and applications

Mock test 8

27 questions
Time allowed 30 minutes
No calculators

Q1   (C4a) What is the percentage of hydrogen in water, atomic mass 18? Give your answer to one decimal place.

(hint: one mole)

Answer [   ]

Q2   (P4c) From a standing start, a Boeing 747 takes off in 40 seconds. If the speed at the point of lift-off is 80 m s^{-1}, what is the average acceleration?

A.   2 m s^{-1}
B.   80 m s^{-2}
C.   20 m s^{-2}
D.   2 m s^{-2}
E.   40 m s^{-1}

(hint: units)

Answer [   ]

Q3   (B2) Identify the correct path for food passing through the digestive system.

A.   Pharynx, oesophagus, stomach, small intestine, large intestine.
B.   Larynx, pharynx, oesophagus, stomach, duodenum, colon.
C.   Pharynx, oesophagus, stomach, large intestine, small intestine.
D.   Larynx, oesophagus, stomach, small intestine, large intestine.
E.   Pharynx, oesophagus, stomach, ileum, duodenum, colon.

Answer [   ]

Q4   (C3a) Which one of the following describes correctly the chemical behaviour of fluorine?

    A.   High electron affinity and a strong reducing agent.
    B.   Most electronegative element and readily oxidized.
    C.   Most electropositive element and readily reduced.
    D.   Most non-metallic element and readily oxidized.
    E.   High electron affinity and a strong oxidizing agent.

Answer

Q5   (P18c,d, 17d) In the circuit shown below, what is the value of the current *I*?

    A.   2 A
    B.   0.5 A
    C.   1 A
    D.   0.4 A
    E.   3 A

(hint: parallel first)

Answer

Q6   (M4a, 5) Calculate $\dfrac{5 + \dfrac{3}{8}}{2 - \dfrac{3}{4}}$

    A.   3.6
    B.   4.0
    C.   4.3
    D.   4.4
    E.   4.8

Answer

Q7   (C4a) Quantitative analysis of a 5 g sample of an unknown compound showed that it contained 2 g of copper. Which of the following could be its chemical formula? (Atomic mass: Cu = 64, C = 12, O = 16, S = 32.)

A. CuO

B. Cu_2O

C. $CuCO_3$

D. $CuSO_4$

E. Cu_2SO_4

(hint: percentage)

Answer [   ]

Q8   (P10e) In a crown green bowling match, a bowl of mass $3M$ strikes a jack of mass M head on.

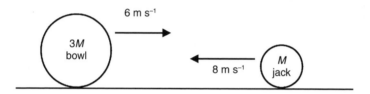

6 m s⁻¹

3M
bowl

8 m s⁻¹

M
jack

Before the collision the bowl has a velocity of 6 m s⁻¹ to the east and the jack has a velocity of 8 m s⁻¹ to the west. If the velocity of the bowl after the collision is 1 m s⁻¹ west, what is the velocity of the jack? Assume that the collision is perfectly elastic.

A. 13 m s⁻¹ east.

B. 13 m s⁻¹ west.

C. 14 m s⁻¹ east.

D. 14 m s⁻¹ west.

(hint: relative velocity; rebound)

Answer [   ]

Q9 (B2) Look at the list (1 to 6) below and then choose the correct path for carbon dioxide leaving the body during exhalation.

1 trachea; 2 bronchioles; 3 bronchi; 4 larynx; 5 pharynx; 6 alveoli.

A. 5, 4, 1, 3, 2, 6
B. 6, 2, 3, 1, 5, 4
C. 6, 2, 3, 1, 4, 5
D. 6, 2, 3, 4, 1, 5
E. 6, 3, 2, 1, 4, 5

Answer

Q10 (M2c, 6c) Calculate the following, giving your answer in scientific notation.

$$\frac{[32 + \log_{10}(10^8)]}{[8 \times 10^{-7} \times (10^3)^4]}$$

Answer

Q11 (P18a,b) Three resistors are connected to a power supply.

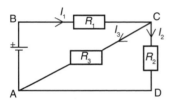

Which of the following statements are true and which are false, according to Kirchhoff's laws?

A. $I_1 = I_2 + I_3$

(hint: node C)

B. $V - I_1R_1 - I_3R_3 = 0$

(hint: loop)

C. $V - I_1R_1 + I_2R_2 = 0$

(hint: Kirchhoff?)

D. $V - I_1R_1 - I_2R_2 - I_3R_3 = 0$

(hint loop?)

A. = ·······
B. = ·······
C. = ·······
D. = ·······

Q12 (C6a) A mouthwash contains 0.2% w/w sodium fluoride. What is the concentration of the fluoride ion in parts per million (ppm) if sodium fluorid is 45% fluoride ion by weight? (Per cent w/w = g/100 g water; ppm = g/million g water.)

A. 45 ppm
B. 450 ppm
C. 90 ppm
D. 900 ppm

Answer [   ]

Q13 (B8(1)) If brown eyes (B) are dominant and blue eyes (b) are recessive, what is the probability that a child will inherit blue eyes if it has a heterozygous mother and a father who has homozygous brown- and blue-eyed parents?

A. 25 per cent
B. 33.3 per cent
C. 50 per cent
D. 75 per cent
E. 100 per cent

(hint: i) father; ii) Punnett square father/mother)

Answer [   ]

Q14 (C5i, 6a,b) Choose the correct word or term (labelled A to K) from the list below to match each numbered space (i to v) in the following text. Some words or terms may be used more than once or not at all.

A = acid; B = base; C = salt; D = 0; E = turns litmus red; F = 7;
G = compound; H = 12; I = ion; J = turns litmus blue; K = 13.

Sodium hydroxide is a strong [...i...]. A 0.01 molar solution has a pH of [...ii...] and [...iii...]. If 100 ml of the solution is titrated against 25 ml of 0.02 molar sulphuric acid the products are a [...iv...] and water; the final pH is [...v...].

i   = ...
ii = ...
iii = ...
iv = ...
v   = ...

Q15 (P17a,b) The diagram shows the position of two positively charged points, 1C and 2C (ie 2 × C) in a grid. In which square does the electric field have the greatest magnitude?

A. i
B. ii
C. iii
D. iv
E. v

(hint: inverse square; vectors)

Answer [   ]

Q16 (B8(2)) A mother expressing an X-linked dominant disease (A) and a father not expressing the disease have one affected son, one unaffected son and one unaffected daughter. Which of the following statements is true?

A. The father is X^AY
B. The mother is X^aX^a
C. The father is X^aY
D. The father is X^aY^A
E. No child is homozygous

(hint: female/male Punnett square; X^A male?)

Answer [   ]

Q17   (C10c) Choose the correct word or term (labelled A to J) from the list below to match each numbered space (i to v) in the following text. Some words or terms may be used more than once or not at all.

A = freezing; B = longest; C = evaporation; D = hydrocarbon; E = condensing; F = volatile; G = least; H = most; I = smallest; J = distillation.

In fractional [...i...] crude oil is separated into fractions. The [...ii...] molecules rise the highest up the tower before [...iii...]. The [...iv...] molecules are the [...v...] flammable and have the lowest boiling point.

i   = ...

ii = ...

iii = ...

iv = ...

v   = ...

Q18   (P19d) The transformer shown below has an output rated at 240 volts and 7.5 amperes. What voltage and current are required at the primary coil?

Primary coil   Secondary coil

A.   60 V, 15 A
B.   120 V, 30 A
C.   240 V, 15 A
D.   120 V, 15 A
E.   360 V, 50 A

(hint: power)

Answer ☐

Q19   (M11) If $y = 0$ when $x = 2$ or -2, what is the value of y when $x = 0$?

    A. +4

    B. −4

    C. +2

    D. −2

    E. 0

(hint: two brackets)

Answer [   ]

Q20   (C7iii) The pH of blood is maintained at 7.4 by the carbonic acid hydrogen carbonate ion buffer as follows:

$$CO_2 + H_2O = H^+ + HCO_3^-.$$

What is the normal response to an increase in carbon dioxide levels in the blood?

    A. The equilibrium shifts to the right and the pH rises.

    B. The equilibrium shifts to the right and the pH falls.

    C. The equilibrium shifts to the right and the pH is unchanged.

    D. The equilibrium shifts to the left and the pH rises.

Answer [   ]

Q21   (B6) Identify the substances i, ii and iii corresponding with the dominant transport processes for molecules passing through the nephron of a normal kidney.

	Transport process		
	Filtration	Re-absorption	Secretion
i	YES	NO	YES
ii	NO	NO	NO
iii	YES	YES	NO

    A. i = glucose; ii = creatinine; iii = protein.

    B. i = creatinine; ii = protein; iii = urea.

    C. i = protein; ii = salt; iii = glucose.

    D. i = creatinine; ii = protein; iii = glucose.

    E. i = urea; ii = protein; iii = creatinine.

Answer [   ]

Q22   (M9a, e) The area of circle A is 16 times that of circle B, which is nine times that of circle C. If the diameter of circle A is 6 cm, what is the diameter of circle C?

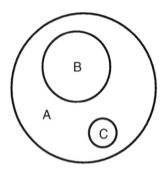

A.   0.25 cm
B.   0.5 cm
C.   0.75 cm
D.   1.0 cm
E.   1.2 cm

Answer

Q23   (B7). Two haploid gametes fertilize to give a diploid zygote that replicates by mitosis to give two identical daughter cells. How many copies of each chromosome are present in a daughter cell when the cells separate at the end of mitosis?

A.   0
B.   1
C.   2
D.   4
E.   8

Answer

Q24 (C9) The apparatus below shows the electrolysis of a dilute solution of sulphuric acid using carbon (inert) electrodes.

Choose the correct word or term (labelled A to H) from the list below to match each numbered space (i to v) in the following text. Some words may be used more than once or not at all.

A = hydrogen sulphide; B = decreases; C = remains the same; D = oxygen; E = twice; F = hydrogen; G = increases; H = half.

The gas discharged at the anode is [...i...] and the gas discharged at the cathode is [...ii...]. The volume of gas at the anode is [...iii...] the volume of gas at the cathode. The pH of the solution [...iv...] and the concentration of the solution [...v...] as the electrolysis progresses.

i   = ...

ii = ...

iii = ...

iv = ...

v   = ...

Q25 (P17d) The charge (Q) in coulombs stored by a capacitor C is given by the formula $Q = CV$ where C is in farads and V in volts. How long will it take to charge a 0.1 F capacitor with a 12 V power supply and a 100 mA charging current?

A. 0.12 s
B. 1.2 s
C. 12 s
D. 120 s
E. 1200 s

(hint: amps: charge s^{-1})

Answer [   ]

Q26 (M10, 11) If $y^2(x^2 - 2x + 1) = 9x^2 + 6x + 1$, what is y in terms of x?

A. $y = 9x^2 + 6x + 1$
B. $y = x^2 + 3x + 1$
C. $y = (3x + 1)(3x - 1)$
D. $y = (3x + 1)/(x - 1)$
E. $y = (3x + 1)/x$

Answer [   ]

Q27 (C9, P14a, P15) The graph shows the time–temperature curve of a liquid when cooled at atmospheric pressure.

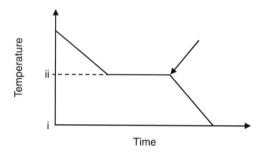

Which of the following statements are true and which are false?

Answer

A. Two phase changes take place.
B. The temperature remains constant during solidification.
C. All the liquid has solidified at the point shown by the arrow.
D. Adding impurities to the liquid will increase ii.
E. The melting and freezing points are the same.

Section 3 Writing task

Mock test 9

Choose one question
Time allowed 30 minutes; you have one side of A4 paper
No dictionaries

1. Not everything that can be counted counts and not everything that counts can be counted (Albert Einstein)

What do you think the author is implying by this statement? Write a unified essay, giving examples that explore the validity of the statement or otherwise.

2. The art of medicine consists in amusing the patient while nature cures the disease (Voltaire, 1694–1778)

What does the author mean by this statement and does it have any relevance today? Advance an argument that reconciles the art of medicine, as you see it, with the ability of nature to cure disease.

3. Education is what remains after one has forgotten what was learned in school (Albert Einstein)

What do you understand by the above statement? Develop an argument that both advances the statement and refutes it?

4. A person may cause evil to others not only by his actions but by his inaction, and in either case he is justly accountable to them for the injury (John Stuart Mill)

What is the author claiming? Develop a balanced argument describing when this might be true, and examples which refute the claim.

Section 1 Aptitude and skills

Mock test 10

35 questions
Time allowed one hour
No calculators

Q1.   If Johnny does not eat a big lunch, he will feel alert at work. If he feels alert at work, he will make fewer errors in typing emails and it will be easier to communicate with his team. If it is easy to communicate with his team, their productivity will increase.

Which is the safest conclusion drawn if the above information is correct?

A.   If Johnny has made more errors in his emails, he will have eaten a big lunch.
B.   If Johnny has lunch, he will not eat a big one.
C.   If Johnny does not feel alert at work, he will make more errors.
D.   If productivity of his team does not increase, Johnny will have communicated with them badly.
E.   If Johnny does not feel alert at work, he will have eaten a big lunch.

Answer ▭

Q2   According to the results of last year's medical school applications at a particular university, 520 students applied, and the university board considered activities of key importance: Voluntary work, hospital work experience and studying abroad. The following are statements about those students:

i)   210 had undertaken voluntary work
ii)   140 had done hospital work experience
iii)   80 had studied abroad
iv)   none had undertaken all three
v)   20 had both voluntary work and hospital experience
vi)   40 had studied abroad and also done hospital work experience
vii) 30 had done voluntary work and studied abroad

Calculate the number of students who did not have any of the three key activities in their application.

Answer ▭

Q3 A group of football players discuss the world's best professional players, and make the following four statements about their group:

i)   No midfielders are fans of Ronaldo, and all midfielders are fans of Robben.
ii) Some strikers are fans of Ronaldo, and some like Bale.
iii) All defenders are fans of Neymar, and some are fans of Robben.
iv) All players are fans of Messi.

Which one of the following statements must be true:

A. Some midfielders are fans of three players.
B. Some strikers are fans of both Ronaldo and Bale.
C. Some defenders are fans of three players.
D. Some midfielders are fans of Bale.
E. Some strikers are fans of Messi, but not Ronaldo or Bale.

Answer _____

Q4 Two colleagues drive to work, each from a distance of 40 miles. Jimmy arrives 14 minutes ahead of Coleen, who had only travelled 33 miles by the time he arrived. Assuming they both drive at a constant velocity, how long did it take Jimmy to arrive at work?

A. 50 minutes
B. 55 minutes
C. 1 hour
D. 1 hour 10 minutes
E. 1 hour 20 minutes

Answer _____

Q5   Complaints against junior doctors mostly come in the area of technical procedures, such as intravenous injections. These claims make up over 60 per cent
of the complaints. In medical school, trainees are taught how to administer
intravenous injections on plastic models and dummies rather than live
patients. Of course, the lack of practice in handling living, breathing humans
means that once a doctor is released onto the wards, he does not have
adequate practical experience. In order to reduce the amount of complaints
about technical procedures, medical schools should incorporate live-patient
training as part of the curriculum, such that junior doctors would not be
qualified until they had appropriate experience.

Which of the following, if true, would weaken the above argument?

i)   Complaints are lowest amongst graduates from schools incorporating
mixed dummy and live-patient training in procedures.

ii) Complaints occur more frequently because junior doctors look young
and therefore inexperienced, making patients uneasy.

iii) Many junior doctors who have complaints made against them in
technical procedures have significant on-the-job experience of
administering such procedures.

A. i only
B. ii only
C. iii only
D. i and ii
E. i and iii

Answer [   ]

Q6   In order to keep ahead of inflation, a prudent sweetshop owner increases his
prices on sherbet by 6 per cent each year. If he currently charges 50 pence
per bag of sherbet (40 grams), and the average customer takes 1.2 kg per
year, how much will they be paying for their year's supply in 3 years' time?

A. £17.87
B. £18.23
C. £19.17
D. £20.21
E. £21.96

Answer [   ]

Q7 Encouraging our children to play video games is the best way to improve the fine-motor skills of future surgeons and pilots. Studies in both fields have demonstrated that the high levels of hand-eye coordination and quick responses required by video games enhance performance of these skills in game players compared to those who have not played games before. Modern games are not a 'waste of time' as some parents think. They are deep, enriching experiences whose multiplayer elements allow the further development of teamwork and communication; important elements of both clinical and aviation professions.

Which one of the following identifies a weakness in the above argument?

A. It assumes that teamwork and communication skills are vital in these professions
B. It ignores the possibility that children play games to pass time rather than learn skills
C. It assumes that children lack hand-eye coordination and quick responses
D. It ignores the possible effects of other activities on fine-motor skill development

Answer ⬚

Q8 The race for the title of 'Best Film' at the Oscars had four potential candidates receiving votes from the Academy. 'Fixback Hill' won 36 votes, and 'Defrosted' garnered half of this amount. 'The Queen's Talk' won 27 votes. 'Totonic' received 25 per cent of the votes.

What was the difference between 1st and 2nd place?

A. 5 votes
B. 6 votes
C. 7 votes
D. 8 votes
E. 9 votes

Answer ⬚

Q9 At the kitchens of a famous bakery, trainee chefs are able to make 20 cakes or 45 cookies per day. To cater for a large wedding of a sweet-toothed bride, 200 cakes and 360 cookies are required, with a deadline of 3 days. What is the minimum number of trainee chefs needed in the kitchen?

A. 3
B. 4
C. 5
D. 6
E. 7

Answer [   ]

Questions 10 and 11 refer to the following information:

Dating and romantic relationships are very complex, and demand a great deal of time, effort and money in order to be successful. Biologists have taken a scientific approach to this problem, learned from the mating patterns of butterflies. Pheromones are microscopic airborne chemical transmitters which are released by butterflies during mating season. Female butterflies find their way towards males by following the concentration gradient, which is at its maximum when nearest the male. In addition to being a direction device, however, it has an effect on the behaviour of the female butterfly, making them more docile and relaxed, allowing the male to mate more easily.

The search for the human pheromone has been remarkable only in its lack of success, until recently. A chemical developed by geneticists known only as QI847, has been shown to have a pheromone-like effect on females which alters their relaxation status, as measured by brainwave activity, pulse and respiration rate. It created a wave of excitement in the business community, and indeed QI847 was created and sold illegally before clinical trials have been completed. It is used by males to attract females, but as we know from research on other relaxant drugs, high levels of exposure can induce heart conditions including arrhythmias where the slowing of the heart causes it to contract in a mis-coordinated fashion. In extreme cases, this has resulted in death. It is therefore hugely irresponsible of the illegal users to expose members of the public to the potentially deadly risks for their own selfish gains.

Q10 Which of the following, if true, represents a flaw in the above argument?

 A. Pheromones occur in primate species which share greater than 99.9 per cent of our DNA and cause no harm to exposed humans.

 B. One of the development scientists of QI847 must have been involved in its illegal release before clinical trial.

 C. The dosage of QI847 available is too low to elicit a response in females.

 D. Brainwave activity is not a reliable measure of relaxation as it differs too greatly between individuals.

 E. Policy preventing the use of drugs before clinical trial data can be enforced by law.

Answer _____

Q11 Which of the following represents a key assumption in the above passage?

 A. The use of pheromones as a direction device is not as important as its effect on behaviour.

 B. Aggressive or agitated partners are more difficult to mate with.

 C. Airborne chemical transmitters need to be microscopic in size in order to reach further distances.

 D. The only cause of arrhythmias in the heart is mis-coordination of contraction.

 E. The type of humans who would use male pheromones are irresponsible.

Answer _____

Q12 One year, a GP consortium decides to reduce the budget for a hospital department by one eighth, to allocate elsewhere. The following year, due to government cuts, all departments receive a 10 per cent reduction. However, the next year a new Secretary of Health is selected, and promises to return the department's budget back to their original levels 2 years ago.

How much does the department's budget need to increase to achieve this aim?

 A. 25 per cent
 B. 26 per cent
 C. 27 per cent
 D. 28 per cent
 E. 29 per cent

Answer _____

Q13   Educational institutions have embraced a culture of creativity in both its staff and their environment. One university has recently employed an award-winning architect to redesign the classrooms, lecture halls and library of the campus, aiming to improve student academic performance. Studies have shown that students benefit the most from collaborative work. Collaboration between students can involve complex methods, including a mix of social media, face-to-face speaking, tablets and mobile devices. Sufficient space is considered to be a key factor in face-to-face interaction, whereas accessibility to power plugs and display screens are critical in electronic collaboration. The architect will incorporate geometric patterns to maximize spacing, and a large number of power plugs near multiple display screens to give enhanced collaborative potential.

What assumption is made by the university in its choice of architectural redesign of the campus?

A.   The architect understands the studying patterns of university students.
B.   The selection of good students for entry to university is more important than campus architecture in determining academic performance.
C.   Academic performance will improve with collaboration.
D.   Students may crowd around display screens, improving electronic learning but impeding face-to-face interaction.
E.   There are several key factors determining the success of collaborative work.

Answer [   ]

Questions 14 and 15 refer to the following information:

An office worker in London attempts to describe his lunch habits over the course of an average four-week period. He states the following information:

i)   On a normal day he will randomly eat either only one sandwich or only one taco at lunchtime with equal chance

ii)   He works 5 days a week

iii)   When he goes to the gym, he randomly eats either 2 tacos or 2 sandwiches with equal chance.

iv)   Every other Monday, there is a Mexican day where he overrides any other behaviour and will eat 5 tacos.

He goes to the gym twice a week on Tuesday and Thursday.

Q14   Assuming the working week starts on Monday and ends on Friday, what is the minimum amount of tacos he could possibly eat in four working weeks?

A.   10
B.   15
C.   20
D.   25
E.   28

Answer

Q15   What is the number of tacos that he will eat in 4 weeks if the random events occur at exactly 50 per cent each?

Answer

Questions 16 to 18 refer to the following passage:

The Large Hadron Collider (LHC) has been the subject of a number of controversial experiments in recent years, with varying degrees of success.

The first is the hunt for the so-called Higgs Boson particle. Unlike all of the other particles which scientists know to make up matter, the presence of this particle has yet to be detected. It is theorized to the 'mass-giving' particle of matter, which is responsible for effects such as gravity. There is now an abundance of data which points to its probable existence, so much so that scientists are almost certain of it, and in reporting to the public, we should consider the existence of the Higgs-Boson to be proven.

Ballodinos are named after an eccentric Italian scientist who came up with a theory that quarks can exist in 4 different states; up, down, left and right. Ballodinos are a particle made up of at least 3 types of these quarks, and they have been observed travelling very short distances inside the LHC. The distances are 4.2 microns for those with all 4 quarks, and 2.8 microns for up, down and left quarks, and 3.1 for up, down and right quarks.

The funding for research of these fundamental particles of our existence mostly comes from independent universities, and although the LHC is based on mainland Europe, the Russell Group of Universities from the UK provides a substantial financial contribution. Of the 35 Universities around the world which are helping, the Russell Group makes up 18 of them.

Q16   Which of the following, if true, would strengthen the above argument relating to the existence for the Higgs Boson?

A.   Many previous 'almost certainties' for scientists turned out to be true.
B.   Academic certainty in physics is based on a sigma 5 significance level.
C.   Unknown to the LHC team, researchers in other laboratories have replicated these results.
D.   This theory can never be conclusively proven or disproven based on the technology available at present.
E.   Reporting of the existence of the Higgs-Boson has already begun in major newspapers.

Answer [   ]

Q17   Based on the information in the above passage alone, which of the following about Balladinos must be true?

A.   There is a 1.4 micron difference between Balladinos with 3 quarks and Balladinos with 4 quarks.
B.   Balladinos with up, left and right quarks travel 3.1 microns.
C.   Balladinos with only right quarks in them travel longer than those with only left quarks.
D.   Balladinos can have more than 4 quarks.
E.   There is a 1.1 micron difference between Balladinos with 4 quarks and Balladinos with an up, down and left quark.

Answer [   ]

Q18   Which of the following statements must be true?

i)   The Russell Group provides the majority of funding for the LHC research
ii)   There are many non-European universities funding LHC research

A.   i only
B.   ii only
C.   i and ii
D.   Neither

Answer [   ]

Questions 19–21 refer to the following information:

A travelling book fair visits various schools around the country, selling revision guides to help students. It visited the smaller towns of Whitby, Ramsgate and Elgin, and the large cities of London and York. Below are their sales figures for 2015:

	Whitby	Ramsgate	Elgin	London	York
Mathematics	12	32	85	162	38
Physics	32	36	20	165	36
Biology	48	41	11	148	34
Chemistry	36	15	84	166	28

Q19 In which school did physics revision guides make up the highest percentage of sales?

A. Whitby
B. Ramsgate
C. Elgin
D. London
E. York

Answer [   ]

Q20 According to the statistics of the authors, reading a revision guide gives a 20 per cent increase on the average mark of students. If we believe the authors, and York has 80 total students whose average mark is 70 per cent in biology, what should the new average mark for the school be, taking into account the effect of the books?

A. 72
B. 74
C. 76
D. 78
E. 80

Answer [   ]

Q21 The authors decide to charge different prices for revisions in different locations, pricing Mathematics at £15 in large cities and £11 in small towns. What was the percentage difference in mathematics revision guide earnings from large cities compared to small towns?

    A. 38
    B. 43
    C. 48
    D. 53
    E. 58

Answer [   ]

Questions 22 and 23 are based on the following statement and reply:

Parent's statement
Students at school are human, and therefore influenced by environmental conditions. One of these is temperature. The rigid conditions of the school uniform in the UK are ridiculous as many institutions require shirt, tie and blazers at all times, regardless of the weather. It is no surprise that my child cannot study as well in school during the summer months. I myself cannot wear a blazer to my office without sweating and discomfort, and being distracted by these very things. Therefore, I support the abandoning of the requirement to wear a blazer to school during the summer.

Headmaster's reply
Our school is proud of our traditions, and I believe this is rightly so. The appearance of our students has an impact on the perception of the school by the public and by important visitors. Rolled-up sleeves and open collars may do for some schools, but not for us. Furthermore, our children live in an era of unprecedented comfort. Learning to struggle through a little suffering will benefit them, by developing mental fortitude and perseverance. Your request for your child not to wear his blazer is unacceptable.

Q22 Which of the following summarizes a critical assumption of the parent's statement?

    A. Dress codes are always enforced in schools.
    B. The suffering of the parent will be mirrored by that of the child.
    C. The UK's weather is consistently hot during the summer months.
    D. Distraction is a direct result of sweating.
    E. Some institutions allow students to dress less formally than others.

Answer [   ]

Q23   Which of the following, if true, would weaken the headmaster's argument?

    A.   The children who study in hot countries perform equally well as UK students in exams.

    B.   Microfibre blazers reduce the amount of extra heat suffered by students compared to normal blazers.

    C.   Dehydration presents a health risk to children who perspire all day.

    D.   A study of children who sat on uncomfortable chairs for a year found they were less attentive and made less effort in class.

    E.   Air conditioning is present throughout the classrooms, hallways and canteens of the school.

                 Answer   ☐

Q24   Competitive sports should be removed from the school curriculum. Children who take part in sports and perform poorly may experience loss of self-esteem and feelings of inferiority in comparison with those who perform better.

    Which of the following is an unstated assumption of the above argument?

    A.   Children are too young to take part in competitive sports.

    B.   Being very good at sport enhances self-esteem and leads to feelings of superiority.

    C.   Competition can be detrimental to psychological health.

    D.   It is not OK to try your best and fail.

    E.   Competitions create winners and losers.

                 Answer   ☐

Q25   Medical school applicants can be split into two groups, A and B. Both groups achieve excellent A-level grades in the subjects with which they are familiar, but group A are better at solving the unfamiliar problems found in the BMAT. Group B can improve their BMAT scores with practice.

    Statement: *Intelligence is largely innate and relatively fixed, whereas 'thinking ability' can be developed.*

    Which of the following best describes how the short statement relates to the passage?

    A.   It has no relevance to the passage.

    B.   It presents a challenge to the passage.

    C.   It supports the passage.

    D.   It explains the poor performance of group B in the BMAT.

    E.   It neither supports nor undermines the passage.

                 Answer   ☐

Questions 26 to 29 refer to the following information:

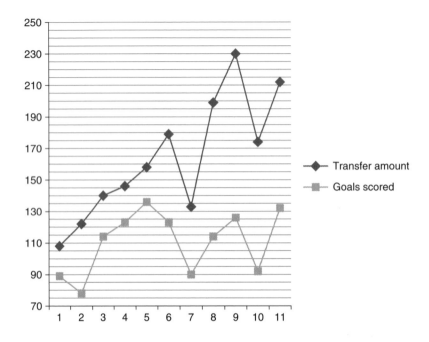

This graph shows the total cost for the top 12 most expensive footballers transferred into the Premier League that season, from year 2001 to 2011. The number of goals scored by those players is also recorded on this graph. **Transfer amount (Y axis) in millions. X axis is year eg 1 = 2001, 2 = 2002 and so on.**

Q26 Which year had the worst goal-to-cost ratio?

    A. 2007
    B. 2008
    C. 2009
    D. 2010
    E. 2011

Answer [   ]

Q27 Which year had the best goal-to-cost ratio?

   A. 2001
   B. 2002
   C. 2003
   D. 2004
   E. 2005

Answer

Q28 In 2008 the top 3 strikers scored 42 per cent of the goals. On average, how many goals were scored by the remaining 9?

   A. 6.9
   B. 7.3
   C. 7.9
   D. 8.4
   E. 9.1

Answer

Q29 Last year, Fernando Torres cost Chelsea £50m and scored only 9 goals. What is the difference between his transfer cost as a percentage of the total compared to his goal contribution as a percentage of the total.

   A. 14.7 per cent
   B. 15.4 per cent
   C. 16.8 per cent
   D. 17.2 per cent
   E. 18.1 per cent

Answer

Q30 Alternative therapies in medicine cover a wide range, including everything from homeopathy, herbal medicine, acupuncture and crystal therapy. Some groups of doctors are against using such treatments on principle: they do not have a clear scientific basis or strong history of clinical trials which demonstrate their effectiveness on patients. Others perceive such therapies in a different light: they may have been passed down from centuries of culture and history, and of course, they argue, that such practices would simply have died out if they did not actually work. Their lack of formal evidence, as undertaken in large studies and published in medical journals, is irrelevant, when you consider the centuries of adoption and refinement which alternative therapies come from. However, the culture of medicine today is one of evidence-based practice and one must rely on scientific trial data above all else. Therefore, alternative therapies should not be used by responsible medical doctors.

Which of the following statements, if true, would provide the strongest support for the above argument?

A. There is an increasing body of clinical trials in therapies such as acupuncture which support its use scientifically.
B. A landmark legal case against a fraudulent homeopathy was recently won in the US.
C. Large clinical trials are themselves affected by deliberate error or bias.
D. The practice of alternative therapies persists because of culture rather than effectiveness.
E. Different alternative therapies have different levels of effectiveness and therefore should not simply be treated the same.

Answer [   ]

Q31 What is the next number in this sequence?

1

11

21

1211

111221

A. 111122
B. 312211
C. 131221
D. 223311
E. 311132

Answer [   ]

Questions 32 and 33 refer to the following information:

Comic conventions attract hundreds of thousands of fans worldwide. Why is this the case? They expend tremendous time, energy and money on dressing up as their favourite characters, a practice known as 'cosplay' (short for costume-play). It seems to many that this is a ridiculous waste of their lives. No doubt their efforts and attention to detail are impressive, but why not put these traits to good use as a St John's Ambulance volunteer or helping in a soup kitchen?

Talking to the fans, however, reveals a deeper level of significance to the individuals' lives. Many describe their interests as niche, and having the experience of being made fun of in schools or in their community. A convention is an area where they can get together and enjoy their mutual enjoyment of a comic, movie or game in a safe environment. Many make friends, and enjoy a sense of escapism from the mundanity of the real world. One fan described her inspiration of playing Japanese anime character *Amane Misa:* 'I've been captivated by the dual personality of Amane, who starts off as an evil protagonist but later overcomes her poignant past to find her true self. Amane reminds me of myself and her courage makes me feel that I too can overcome any hurdles at school.' The truth behind comic convention fans' attendance is that they are seeking inspiration as much as alleviating their loneliness.

Q32 Which one of the following is the best expression of the main conclusion in the above argument?

A. Fruitful pursuits such as volunteer work are more important than those of pure entertainment.
B. Individual fans may find inspiration from single characters or comics.
C. Convention attendees should not be considered to be wasting their time.
D. Feelings of loneliness and seeking inspiration motivate fans' attendance at comic conventions.
E. Comic conventions provide an escape from reality.

Answer ⬚

Q33 Which of the following, if true, would most seriously weaken the above argument?

A. Studies show that comic convention fans are more susceptible to advertising.

B. The demographics of attendees show greater than 60 per cent male attendance.

C. Convention organizers report serious incidents of harassment and violence at some events.

D. St John's ambulance volunteers are also motivated by finding company and friends in their activities.

E. Comic fans are reported to exhibit mild versions of obsessive or addictive behaviour.

Answer [   ]

Questions 34 and 35 refer to the following information:

When a company forms, ownership is divided amongst the founders and is called equity. Individuals receive a percentage of equity based on their contributions to 5 areas; ideas, commitment, special skills, network and finance (money they put forward). Each category is scored out of 100 and weighted out of 10. The equity allocated is the weighted score of the individual divided by the sum of the weighted scores of all the founders. Below represents an equity calculation between three owners.

Category	Weight	Scores				
		Chris	Steph	Arthur		
Idea	2	100	0	0		
Commitment	10	60	15	15		
Special Skills	5	80	50	50		
Network	4	20	80	50		
Finance	6	80	20	0		

Q34   Assuming the money Chris put forward was $150,000, how much did Steph
contribute?

A. $32,000
B. $35,500
C. $37,500
D. $40,000
E. $42,500

Answer

Q35   How much equity should Arthur get?

A.   16.50 per cent
B.   16.85 per cent
C.   17.45 per cent
D.   18.25 per cent
E.   18.75 per cent

Answer

Section 2 Scientific knowledge and applications

Mock test 11

27 questions
Time allowed 30 minutes
No calculators

Q1   Some pathogens have significant resistance to human immune processes by developing the following characteristics:

i)   Surface proteins to avoid ingestion.
ii)   Envelopes which are resistant to antibodies.
iii)   Production of toxins.

Which of the above would be effective against the actions of white blood cells?

A.   i only
B.   ii only
C.   iii only
D.   i and ii only
E.   ii and iii only
F.   All of the above

Answer   _____

Q2   Which of the following are monoprotic acids?

i)   Citric acid
ii)   Hydrocholoric acid
iii)   Nitric acid

A.   i only
B.   ii only
C.   iii only
D.   i and iii only
E.   ii and iii only
F.   None of the above

Answer   _____

Q3   Justin B is driving a car at 10m/s when the engine suddenly fails. The car experiences a deceleration of –2m/s². Orlando steps into the road 40 metres from the point where the engine fails. How close does the car come to hitting Orlando?

A. 3m
B. 6m
C. 10m
D. 12m
E. 15m

Answer

Q4   Simplify

$$\frac{5x+15}{x^2-9} \times \frac{y-4}{4-y}$$

A. $5/(3-x)$
B. $3/xy$
C. $-5/(x+3)$
D. $5/(4-yx)$
E. $X/4\sqrt{y}$

Answer

Q5   Which of the following correctly describes the sequence of events that result in the transmission of a signal at a synapse between neurons?

i)   Action potential is triggered in the second neuron.
ii)   Action potential arrives at first neuron.
iii) Transmitter molecules are released from the pre-synaptic bulb of the first neuron.
iv) Transmitter molecules are produced by the pre-synaptic bulb of the first neuron.
v)   Transmitter molecules diffuse across the synapse.

A. i → iv → iii → v → ii
B. ii → iv → iii → v → i
C. iii → ii → iv → ii → v
D. iv → ii → iii → v → i
E. ii → iii → iv → v → i

Answer

Q6   A hotel spa is set up so that one loudspeaker plays music in a room, and another plays music underwater such that they can be heard in a swimming pool. The speed of sound is 340 m/s in air, but 1400 m/s in water. If both loudspeakers reverberate at 500hz, what is the difference in wavelength between the sound in water and that in the air in centimetres?

A.   212
B.   238
C.   280
D.   320
E.   352

Answer

Q7   In the following fairground game, the sequence of numbers is used as a 'board', whereupon players can attempt to drop a ball on a specific digit. Due to some variation, the ball has a chance of landing on the target itself, or one digit to the right or left of it.

7   8   4   9   2   5   6   10

The first and last digit of the sequence cannot be selected as targets.

Given that the ball has an equal probability of landing on the target, left or right, which two digits can be selected which have an equal probability of the same score?

Answer

Q8   Regarding the homeostasis of blood, if the following conditions were present:

Greater reabsorption of water and glucose in the kidneys and increased blood level of glucose.

Which of the following would result in the above conditions?

i)   Diabetes Mellitus
ii)   Damage to the nephrons
iii) Dehydration

A. i only
B. ii only
C. iii only
D. i and ii only
E. i and iii only
F. ii and iii only
G. None of the above

Answer

Q9   A government issues guidelines for the maximum safe levels of radiation in a single dose as follows:

(all figures given in micro-sieverts [µSv])

	Any radiation type stopped by skin	Any radiation type which penetrates the skin	Any radiation source which is inhaled or ingested
Adult	3.1×10^4	2.4×10^2	310
Child (under 18)	2.3×10^4	8.6×10^3	210

Which of the following situations would be considered safe under these guidelines?

i)   Adult exposed to 220 µSv of gamma radiation in a radiology department.
ii)   Child holding a 7500 µSv cube of Strontium-90 (beta radiation source).
iii) Adult exposed to 3×10^4 µSv of alpha-emitting radon gas.

A. i only
B. ii only
C. iii only
D. i and ii
E. ii and iii
F. None of the above

Answer

Q10   Assuming all of the below undergo a decomposition reaction, which 2 compounds will produce the products which can react in a 2:1 ratio to form a salt?

i) NH_4Cl
ii) H_2O_2
iii) $CaCO_3$
iv) Na_2CO_3

A. i and ii
B. i and iii
C. i and iv
D. ii and iii
E. ii and iv
F. iii and iv

Answer

Q11   Regarding the following sequence of numbers:

1, 2, 4, 6, 10, 12, x

What is the next number in the sequence?

Answer

Q12   The game Jenga involves stacking wooden rectangles on top of each other, with a maximum of 3 rectangles per layer. This stacking continues until the whole column loses balance, and falls over. If each of the wooden rectangles weighs 120 grams, what is the velocity of the rectangle immediately before it impacts the ground if the height of the stack is 2 metres when it falls? (Ignore air resistance, g = 10m/s²)

A. $\sqrt{28}$ m/s
B. $\sqrt{34}$ m/s
C. $\sqrt{40}$ m/s
D. $\sqrt{48}$ m/s
E. $\sqrt{52}$ m/s

Answer

Q13 Genetically modified crops are usually designed to:

   i)   Have more resistance to insect attacks
   ii) Have more resistance to insecticides
   iii) Have no effect on insect populations
   iv) Be less affected by herbicides
   v)   Have increased crop yields

   Which of the above statements are true?

   A. i, ii and v
   B. i, iii and v
   C. i, iii and iv
   D. ii, iii, iv and v
   E. i, ii, iv and v
   F. i, iii, iv and v
   G. All of the above

   Answer _____

Q14 A light bulb has a resistance of 500 ohms, and is supplied with a current of 500 milliamperes running through it. It emits a total of 20 watts of useful light energy. What is its efficiency in terms of producing light?

   A. 8 per cent
   B. 16 per cent
   C. 34 per cent
   D. 40 per cent
   E. 52 per cent

   Answer _____

Q15 In the case of oil spills at sea, chemical dispersants are used to break up the oil slick by binding to oil particles. One newly developed chemical dispersant has the following characteristics; it binds with the highest affinity to highest carbon-carbon bonds; triple, then double, then single. Which of the following compounds would be dispersed at the fastest rate?

   A. Propane
   B. Benzene
   C. Propene
   D. Polyethene
   E. Propyne

   Answer _____

Q16 The following statements relate to a simple reflex arc:

i) Sensory neurones synapse with relay neurones in the central nervous system.

ii) Relay neurones synapse with motor neurones outside of the central nervous system.

iii) The effector is a muscle.

Which of the above must be true?

A. i only
B. ii only
C. iii only
D. i and ii only
E. ii and iii only
F. i and iii only
G. All of the above

Answer

Q17 Simplify:

$$\frac{3x^2+17x+20}{3x^2+23x+30}$$

Answer

Q18 With regards to electricity:

i)   Increasing voltage reduces energy loss in transmission through cables for a given power.
ii) Step up transformers have high numbers of primary turns relative to secondary.
iii) Electricity for households is billed as energy transferred measured in kW.
iv) Field strength of a magnetic field generated from a current passing through a wire is proportional to the current from the wire.

Which of the above are true?

A.   i and ii
B.   i and iii
C.   i, ii and iii
D.   i and iv
E.   ii and iv
F.   iii and iv
G.   ii, iii and iv
H.   All of the above

Answer ⬚

Q19 Which of the following proteins found in the body, function best in the corresponding conditions?

1	2	3
Higher temperature	Higher concentration	Higher concentration
Low pH	Higher temperature	High pH

A.   Protease, insulin, antibodies
B.   Amylase, antibodies, protease
C.   Protease, antibodies, lipase
D.   Insulin, protease, amylase
E.   Lipase, insulin, protease

Answer ⬚

Q20   A chemist was given aluminium from a disreputable source, and decides to test its purity. He reacts a sample of it with an excess of copper(II) sulphate solution, 4.0 g of aluminium is reacted and 0.6 g of copper metal is formed. What percentage of the sample is aluminium?

A.   34%
B.   38%
C.   42%
D.   46%
E.   52%

Answer [   ]

Q21   Regarding the conduction of thermal energy:

i)   The human perception of an item feeling warm or cold is in part due to its conductivity than its actual temperature.
ii)   Heat cannot spontaneously go from a colder location to a hotter one.
iii) Microwaves heat food by causing rotation of polar water molecules within them.
iv)   Frozen food heats less well by microwaves than unfrozen food as it has less water.

Which of the above are true?

A.   i and ii
B.   ii and iii
C.   ii and iv
D.   i and iv
E.   i, ii and iii
F.   i, ii and iv
G.   ii, iii and iv
H.   All of the above

Answer [   ]

Q22   Regarding meiosis in humans:

      i)   Meiosis produces diploid cells

      ii)   Meiosis occurs after puberty

      iii)   Meiosis only occurs when reproducing

Which of the above are true?

    A.   i only

    B.   ii only

    C.   iii only

    D.   i and ii only

    E.   i and iii only

    F.   ii and iii only

    G. None of the above

Answer

Q23   Regarding rates of reaction, which of the following will not result in the increased rate of reaction?

      i)   The temperature is increased

      ii)   The pressure of a reacting gas is increased

      iii)   More solute is applied for a dissolved reactant

      iv)   Dividing solid reactants pieces

      v)   A catalyst is introduced

    A.   i only

    B.   ii only

    C.   iii only

    D.   iv only

    E.   v only

    F.   ii and iv only

    G. ii and v only

Answer

Q24 A sports club constructs a circular jacuzzi of diameter D and depth H. It needs to provide tiling for the walls of this pool. What is the total surface area of this pool which needs tiling?

A. $\pi D^2 + \pi HD$
B. $2\pi DH + \pi D^2$
C. $\pi DH + \pi(D/2)^2$
D. $2\pi DH + \pi(2/D)^2$
E. $\pi DH + \pi D^2$

Answer _____

Q25 The radioactive decay of substance x causes it to form substance y. Below is a graph indicating the remaining amount of substance x at various times:

Time (Minutes)	Substance x (mg)
10	136.5
20	108.5
30	86.0
40	68.3
50	54.1
60	43.0
70	34.1

Calculate the starting amount of substance x

A. 214
B. 202
C. 186
D. 172
E. 154

Answer _____

Q26   A normal light bulb receives a 10 ampere current, and produces 140 joules of light energy per second. A power-saving light bulb receives an 8 ampere current, but produces 320 joules of light energy per second. Both are supplied by a 240 volt system. What is the difference in efficiency between the two types of bulb?

A.   4.5 per cent
B.   7.8 per cent
C.   9.2 per cent
D.   10.9 per cent
E.   14.6 per cent

Answer

Q27   In a game show challenge, a contestant has to run up a 100m slope with an incline of 1 in 10 (for each 10m of distance along, the height is increased by 1m). He starts off carrying 3 blocks of different masses at different points along the way. The contestant weighs 60kg, and drops block A after 20m, block B after 40m and block C after 60m. If block A is 10kg, block B 5kg and block C 2kg, how much work does he undertake in completing the challenge? (Ignore friction, $g = 10m/s^2$)

A.   6520
B.   8400
C.   10890
D.   13040
E.   15390

Answer

Section 3 Writing task

Mock test 12

Choose one question
Time allowed 30 minutes; you have one side of A4 paper.
No dictionaries

1. It is dangerous that science gathers knowledge faster than society gathers wisdom

What do you understand by the terms knowledge and wisdom? Develop a unified argument that contradicts this opinion. To what extent is the statement true? Can you reconcile medicine as both art and science?

2. Medicine sometimes snatches away health, sometimes gives it (Ovid)

Explain what the author is indicating about medicine. Is the order in which he expresses the ideas significant? Construct a balanced argument with supportive examples.

3. The roots of education are bitter, but the fruit is sweet (Aristotle)

What is the author implying in comparing the roots and fruit of education? Can you give examples which support and refute his position on the sweetness and bitterness of these activities? To what extent do you agree with him?

4. Opt-out policy for organ donation should be the norm; you will then have to convince me that after you die, you still do not want to save another's life

What does the author mean by opt-out policy? How might you convince him that after death, you do not want to save another's life? To what extent do you agree with his position?

Section 1 Aptitude and skills

Mock test 13

35 questions
Time allowed one hour
No calculators

Q1   We live in the lie of the 'meritocratic society'. We are told that people can
achieve whatever they like, as long as they work hard. The sky is the limit
when it comes to human potential. You can all be famous, rich, proud achievers. Unfortunately, there is a downside to this philosophy. For those people
who are poor, according to this system, they deserve to be in the position they
are. If successful people succeed due to hard work, the corollary of this is that
those who are unsuccessful are lazy, and deserve their suffering. Therefore,
we should not believe in the lie that our society is meritocratic. People succeed because of factors outside of their own effort, including their parents'
success, country of origin, race and most of all, luck.

Which of the following effectively summarises the conclusion of the passage?

A.   Society unfairly glamorizes the rich, famous or high achievers.
B.   People are poor because they are unwilling to work as hard as successful
people.
C.   Our society should strive to be meritocratic.
D.   Not all people are unsuccessful through their own fault.
E.   Success is a multi-factorial phenomenon.

Answer   ☐

Q2   In a small football league, four teams play each of the other teams just once per season to determine the winner. A win scores 3 points, a draw scores 1 point and a loss scores 0 points. Here is the league table at the end of the season.

Team	Points
Best United	7
Good FC	?
OK Town	3
Terrible City	0

How many points must Good FC have?

A. 3
B. 4
C. 5
D. 6
E. 7

Answer [   ]

Q3   Recent studies have indicated that champagne is less detrimental to the health of drinkers when compared to normal wine. Of course, both products contain alcohol, which is damaging to various parts of the body when consumed in excess. However, wine also requires the inclusion of tannins and sulphides as part of the manufacturing. Due to the unique fermentation process of champagne, which utilises yeast inside the bottles themselves, these chemicals are not needed. In addition, this in-bottle fermentation produces carbon dioxide, and as it dissolves into the liquid, this is what results in the lovely, bubbly champagne in the end. In recent years, champagne has become more popular than wine due to the enjoyment of the bubbly taste.

Sadly, winemakers are starting to use the popularity of champagne to increase their own revenues, by adding carbon dioxide to wine in a number of different ways to also make it bubbly. This may increase the sales of their wine, making it seem similar to champagne, but the presence of tannins and sulphides which are harmful to humans will have a negative impact on the health of the drinking population. We therefore strongly oppose the promotion of this carbonated wine as 'champagne', and discourage its use by everyone. Demand real champagne!

Which of the following can be safely concluded if the passage above is true?

A. The fermentation of wine does not involve yeast, therefore it is not bubbly like champagne unless carbon dioxide is added.
B. Tannins and sulphides represent the main risk when drinking wine, but not champagne.
C. Drinking champagne can be beneficial to health.
D. Carbonating wine is a cheap method of producing champagne.
E. Alcoholic drinks can be harmful to health.

Answer [   ]

Q4   Your friend sends out an invitation to a board game party at his house, but accidentally posts it on his social network publically. As a result, an unknown number of guests arrive. However, they are well behaved and he lets them play.

There is a single board game which takes a maximum of 5 players. Each player must read the rulebook which takes 25 minutes, and only one person can read it at a time. When all players have read the rule book, the game commences, and lasts a total of 15 minutes. During this period, waiting players may read the rulebook. When players finish the game, they leave. If there are not enough players to make a game of 5, the game commences when all remaining players have read the rulebook.

If the party starts at 2pm and the final guests leave at 7.40pm, how many people came to the party?

A. 8
B. 13
C. 15
D. 17
E. 19

Answer [   ]

Questions 5 and 6 refer to the following information:

When students apply for medical school, they are required to write a personal state-ment which acts as an essay discussing their motivations for a career in medicine. In order to facilitate an informed and measured application, students can undertake work experience placements in hospitals. Doctors who come across such students are faced with a dilemma. When they first arrive, often students have a rosy ideal of what the life of a doctor is like: smiling whilst attending to the cares of patients in a pleasant and friendly environment. The truth is far starker. Bodily fluids, odours, angry relatives, long working hours and poor working conditions are often the experience of the doctors' lives. However, when doctors discuss their careers, they are becoming more scrutinized in their feedback, and students are beginning to complain that the doctors are too negative, putting them off from a potential career pursuing medicine. Unfortunately, there appears to be real grounds for avoiding this kind of 'real' feed-back to students. There have been cases where senior doctors receive complaints against their staff on these grounds, and students have been reported as giving up their choice to study medicine. This effect is continuing to the degree that there are recruitment issues for medical staff in the UK. Sadly, it seems that the authentic account and experience of life as a doctor is something for which students are not yet ready to face.

Q5   Which of the following is a principle which could give support to the above argument?

   A.   Medical students should be given a clear understanding of a doctor's life.
   B.   Students who are put off from a medical career early would not have the stamina to finish the difficult course.
   C.   It is important that there are sufficient doctors recruited and trained.
   D.   It is unfair to misrepresent the reality of a medical career to a student.

   Answer [   ]

Q6   Which of the following, if true, represents a weakness in the above argument?

   A.   Some individuals enjoy the challenge of long hours and dealing with dif-ficult relatives.
   B.   Every career has difficult aspects which are not obvious to applicants.
   C.   Informing students of the difficulties of medicine acts as a filter to remove applicants unsuited to ward life.
   D.   Rosy ideals of medical life are often the result of medical school appli-cants having one or more parents being a doctor.

   Answer [   ]

Q7   At the World Cup in Brazil 2014, a third of the incidents involving violence involved groups of fans from a European team which did not qualify past the group stages of the competition.

Which of the following can be safely inferred from this information?

i)   European fans whose team did not qualify past the group stages are more violent than those whose team qualified.

ii)   At least one third of violent incidents involved teams who did not qualify past the group stages.

iii)   The fans whose teams did not qualify past the group stages should be sent home to reduce violent incidents.

A.   i only
B.   ii only
C.   iii only
D.   i and ii only
E.   i and iii only

Answer

Questions 8 to 11 refer to the following information:

Couples head out on a double date to watch a movie at their local cinema. The trailers prior to the film show at 7.35 and the film itself shows at 8pm. They live at the following distances, and use the following methods of transport:

	Method of transport	Average speed (Km/h)	Distance from cinema (Km)
Max	Motorbike	25	12.2
Julie	Walking	3.2	1.1
Agatha	Bus	9.8	3.5
Shane	Car	30	11.5

Q8   Who has the shortest journey time to the cinema?

A.   Max
B.   Julie
C.   Agatha
D.   Shane

Answer [   ]

Q9   The group has decided to meet just in time to catch the trailers. What time does Agatha leave?

A.   7.13 and 24 seconds
B.   7.14 and 30 seconds
C.   7.13 and 36 seconds
D.   7.13 and 40 seconds
E.   7.14 and 38 seconds

Answer [   ]

Q10   Julie leaves on time, but immediately remembers that she hates watching trailers, and decides to walk a bit slower so she arrives *just* in time for the movie instead. At what speed should she walk.

A.   1.3 km / hour
B.   1.4 km / hour
C.   1.5 km / hour
D.   1.6 km / hour
E.   1.7 km / hour

Answer [   ]

Q11   Agatha leaves on time, but takes the bus which, because it is in London, could make her up to 10 minutes early or late. Calculate the difference in average speed between the maximum and minimum in km per hour, including her stationary waiting time.

A.   10.2 km / hour
B.   10.9 km / hour
C.   11.7 km / hour
D.   12.4 km / hour
E.   13.6 km / hour

Answer [   ]

Questions 12 and 13 refer to the following information:

Republic of Widiya is ruled by a great dictator, who has ruled that he will not trade with the corrupt Western Powers.

Their currency is the Dyat, and no other country will accept it apart from North Korean Won, Chinese Ren Min Bi or Jordanian Dinar.

Therefore tourists there are forced to trade currency, currently at the following rate:

	Exchange rate to 1 Dyat
Ren Min Bi	10.6
North Korean Won	30.5
Jordanian Dinar	6.0

Holidaydollar	2.0%	5 Dyat
Travelcash	2.5 %	4 Dyat
Movemoolah	3.1%	No fee
Sunny Exchange	3.0%	1 Dyat
Cashmoney	2.2%	3 Dyat

The calculations are done by taking the commission off from the amount converted to Dyat, and subsequently removing any fee due.

Q12   Who provides the best deal for changing large amounts of currency?

A. Holidaydollar
B. Travelcash
C. Movemoolah
D. Sunny Exchange
E. Cashmoney

Answer [   ]

Q13   How much Dyat would I get if I changed 250 Jordanian Dinar at Cashmoney?

A. 37.75
B. 37.95
C. 38.05
D. 39.50
E. 39.60

Answer [   ]

Q14 Microchips are made of a silicon base with semiconductor materials embedded on them in fine pathways in order to conduct electronic signals. In order for computer technology to continue to advance at its current rate, new ways of minimizing the size of microchips are required. This is due to two reasons. Firstly, the smaller the size of the microchip, the lesser the distance which signals are required to travel. This results in reduced processing times, and faster computers. The second is to do with temperature; when signals are sent at a high rate, electrical potential energy is dissipated as heat. The larger the microchip, the greater the amount of heat, and the more difficult it is to cool the processor. If the processor cannot be cooled sufficiently, it will melt down, and therefore the only way to avoid this in large microchips is to run them slowly. Fortunately, researchers have developed a new method embedding semiconductor materials onto silicon in microscopic amounts. This means that at least for now, the next steps in advancing computer technology and faster microchips are secure.

Which of the following represents a flaw in the above argument?

A. It assumes that processors cannot be cooled by external devices.
B. The cost of the new method of manufacturing has not been considered.
C. It assumes that smaller microchips are always superior to larger ones.
D. It assumes that the method of inscribing can create functional microchips.
E. It assumes that faster microchips are required for advancing computer technology.

Answer _____

Q15 The following table describes the classes of haemorrhage from I–IV, showing the amount of blood lost, the predicted patient response:

Class	Blood loss	Response
I	<15%	Resting heart rate increase by 18 per cent
II	15–30%	Resting heart rate increase by 22 per cent
III	30–40%	Resting heart rate increase by 28 per cent
IV	>40%	Resting heart rate increase by 38 per cent

If the average man has a normal total blood volume of 3.2 litres and resting heart rate of 60, what is his expected heart rate upon losing 600ml of blood?

A. 71
B. 73
C. 75
D. 77
E. 79

Answer [   ]

Questions 16 and 17 refer to the following information:

Repetitive strain injuries of the wrist are defined by suffering chronic pain, and are becoming more widespread with the increasing use of electronic equipment. It comes about by frequent and prolonged motions, typically with the hands, for example in typing, using a computer mouse or in manual tasks such as cooking or construction. Students use laptops more frequently than even 10 years ago, and are now considered to be at serious risk of the disease. According to recent studies, the problem occurs because our tendons are not friction free: they lie within 'sheaths' or containers which are bathed in liquid. This reduces, but does not eliminate the friction, meaning that repeated use leads to increased temperature, wear and tear and eventually inflammation and therefore pain. In order to prevent such problems, doctors are recommending wrist splints which reduce the range of motion, reducing the development of inflammation.

As a result of these studies, students are the latest group which should be recommended these precautionary measures such as splints. Office workers, chefs and even professional sportspeople are already recommended such splints due to their occupations, which almost certainly involve repetitive motions over a prolonged period.

Q16 Which of the following best expresses the main conclusion of the passage?

A. Students should not overuse their laptops.
B. Wrist splits will always prevent inflammation.
C. Office workers usually suffer from repetitive strain injuries.
D. Students should be recommended to wear wrist splints.
E. Friction in the tendon sheaths is the cause of repetitive strain injuries.

Answer [   ]

Q17 Which of the following is a major assumption made by the above passage?

    A. Repetitive strain injuries mainly occur in the upper body.
    B. Inflammation leads to pain.
    C. Students can avoid using laptops by utilising pen and paper.
    D. Wrist splints do not obstruct the day to day activities of wearers.
    E. All people at risk would wear wrist splints if recommended by doctors.

Answer [   ]

Q18 A recently married couple discovered that they each have an expensive interest. The husband enjoys buying antique furniture, and his wife enjoys eating rare truffles. Their habits last year were such that they spent 80 per cent of their total household income on these two luxuries, and the antique furniture contributes to 60 per cent of this.

    If their previous combined income was £110,000 and their absolute expenditure on luxuries remains the same, what percentage of their household income is spent on rare truffles if their income is increased to £140,000?

    A. 25 per cent
    B. 26 per cent
    C. 27 per cent
    D. 28 per cent
    E. 29 per cent

Answer [   ]

Questions 19 and 20 refer to the following information:

One of the most exciting developments in the field of biotechnology is undoubtedly the use of algae to produce biofuels. Algae are hugely common, small plants which live in the sea and survive by photosynthesis. With a surprisingly small amount of genetic modification, these algae can be changed to produce oil instead of carbohydrates, and this oil can be used as a substitute for petroleum in specially modified cars. Imagine what this means. No longer do we need to construct so-called 'large' and expensive solar panels covering one or two square kilometres. Now we could potentially use the sea as our photosynthetic fuel source, and having thousands of square kilometres is a fraction of one per cent of the vast oceans available to us.

Whilst this development is indeed exciting, biofuels are not as environmentally friendly as they are perceived by many to be. The truth is that the combustion of oil in the modified cars still produces carbon dioxide and other greenhouse gases which contribute to global climate change. Simple economics states that the increase in output of an available and cheap fuel will increase demand in commuting, which would in turn have a negative effect on the global climate. Solar panels, whilst less exciting, have less of a carbon footprint in the long term.

Q19 Which of the following can be drawn as a conclusion from the above passage?

    A. Biofuels will provide a greater usable fuel source than solar panels.

    B. The increased use of algae-derived biofuels will cause environmental problems.

    C. Using large areas of sea for algae biofuels may cause marine life imbalance.

    D. Carbon footprint is the key consideration in the economics of fuel sources.

Answer [   ]

Q20 Which of the following, if true, would most significantly support the above passage?

    A. Per square kilometre, solar panels are significantly more efficient at converting solar energy into usable energy.

    B. Genetic modification of rapidly breeding species such as algae can result in damaging the oxygen balance of the ocean.

    C. Industrial processes of manufacture such as sugar refinement and textile production have the largest impact on climate change.

    D. The combustion profile of biofuel has less impact on climate change than those of fossil fuels.

Answer [   ]

Q21   In the UK, there are strict laws governing the conditions under which abortion is legal. These stem from the days of 'back alley' abortions, which used dangerous tools in unsterile environments by untrained staff. In order to prevent the impact of infection and risk to mothers who wanted an abortion, in 1967 the Abortion Act was passed, making it only legal for medical practitioners to perform abortions in certain conditions after 24 weeks gestation, for example risk to the mother or baby, a serious risk of the baby having a severe disease at birth or in pregnancy as a result of sexual assault. As you can imagine, some doctors are against performing abortions on principle, be it religious or philosophical. It is legal for them to conscientiously object and refuse to undertake the abortion themselves. However, even if one doctor objects in this manner, there is nothing preventing you from seeking a second opinion from another doctor. Given the thousands of doctors one might see in the UK, it is impossible not to get an abortion if you try hard enough. Therefore, we can conclude that in the UK at least, if you really want to have an abortion, you can do so regardless of whether the first doctor you see agrees with you or not.

Which of the following represents a flaw in the argument?

A.   An objecting doctor is not obliged to refer you to another doctor.
B.   Many UK doctors are against performing abortions after 24 weeks gestation.
C.   Being pregnant always involves a high risk to the mother's health.
D.   Legal reasons are different from philosophical reasons for objecting to abortions.
E.   Illegal abortions by non-medical staff are still commonplace in the UK.

Answer [   ]

Questions 22 to 25 refer to the following information:

	Single burger	Drink	Fries	Dessert	MEAL DEAL
McColonel	£2.00	£0.90	£0.50	£1.20	£3.68
Burger Ronald	£2.20	£0.60	£0.30	£1.10	£3.20
King Fried Chicken	£3.40	£1.20	£0.90	£1.70	£7.20
Wompy	£2.40	£1.00	£1.00	£1.00	£4.32

	Single burger	Drink	Fries	Dessert
McColonel	320	120	140	200
Burger Ronald	240	150	140	220
King Fried Chicken	480	100	150	220
Wompy	300	120	145	210

A Meal Deal includes a single burger, fries, dessert and drink

Q22 What percentage of calories in the King Fried Chicken meal deal is made up by the fries?

A.   14.2 per cent
B.   14.5 per cent
C.   15.3 per cent
D.   15.7 per cent
E.   16.2 per cent

Answer

Q23 What is the cheapest calorie per cost available between the burgers?

A.   McColonel
B.   Burger Ronald
C.   King Fried Chicken
D.   Wompy

Answer

Q24 Legislation comes in to ensure that meal options must be available with a salad. What is the percentage decrease of the calories per meal if fries were replaced with an 80 calorie salad in the McColonel meal?

A. 8 per cent
B. 9 per cent
C. 10 per cent
D. 12 per cent
E. 13 per cent

Answer

Q25 'Live below the line' is a campaign in which people live on a minimal amount of money for a week to raise awareness of starvation. What is the most economical way to gain the calories from the options below?

A. KFC Drink
B. KFC Dessert
C. Wompy Burger
D. Wompy Drink
E. Wompy Dessert

Answer

Q26 Magicians use our limited abilities to focus attention to take advantage of us for our own entertainment. Consider the senses involved in a magic show: sight, sound and touch. How does a magician appear to magically remove the watch from a guest? By misdirecting their attention to one of these senses, for example by waving a wand, the sensation of touch in having your watch removed is lessened. Young people are more vulnerable to this type of mis-direction as their bodies have not adapted to different stimuli over the years. The older you are, the less 'new' a sight, sound or touch is, and therefore the less distracting you will find it. This is the reason why young people enjoy magic shows more than older people; they are biologically more susceptible to its methods.

Which of the following identifies a weakness in the above argument?

i)   Older people have lower attention spans than young people.
ii) Magic shows tend to be youth orientated in their style and presentation.
iii) Different individuals find stimuli of certain senses more distracting than others.

A. i only
B. ii only
C. iii only
D. i and ii only
E. ii and iii only
F. i, ii and iii

Answer

Q27 The focus of the Centre for Disease Control (CDC) in the USA has always been to save the greatest amount of lives. Since this is its priority, the focus should always be on communicable diseases or epidemics. These are events in which thousands of people die due to a single source: as recently as 2013 an outbreak of cyclosporiasis devastated the community of East Texas, killing over 1670 people in the course of three months. If you compare this to deadly but non-communicable diseases such as stroke, you can see that the obsession with such diseases is ill-advised. Stroke can only kill one individual and cannot be transmitted. Epidemics like swine flu, legionella and cyclosporiasis kill communities, as we continue to see to this very day.

Which of the following two statements are flaws of the above argument?

A. The difference in the cost of treating communicable diseases and individual diseases is not considered.
B. The relative frequencies of the diseases are not considered.
C. The difference in disease management in different states is not considered.
D. The role of non-medical intervention in epidemics is not considered.
E. The way in which epidemics and individual diseases are portrayed in the media impacts their public perception.

Answer

Q28 Which one of the following letters will not look correct if it is turned upside down and reflected in a mirror?

B C I E X S

Answer [   ]

Q29 What is the missing letter in the table below?

?	B	D	C
C	A	B	F
B	E	C	B
D	D	C	A

Answer [   ]

Q30 Entrepreneurs who have million-dollar businesses before the age of 30 all have one underlying characteristic: excellence in the skills of information technology (IT). The most successful cases in recent years are Lu Zhang from China and Iswal Randi from India, both of whose parents are IT consultants themselves, and as a result exposed their children to coding data from a young age. Parents who wish their child to be skilled IT entrepreneurs should also train their children in IT skills from a young age.

Which of the following represents an assumption made by the above passage?

A. China and India are upcoming economies which are easier to succeed in as an entrepreneur.
B. IT skills are the only determinant of being a successful entrepreneur.
C. Exposing children to coding data from a young age has a direct impact on their IT skills.
D. Children from India and China are more talented in IT skills.
E. Multi-million dollar business owners before the age of 30 differ significantly from those who own them after the age of 30.

Answer [   ]

Q31 The World Health Organisation (WHO) performs studies of the largest scale, involving the equivalent of the entire populations of many countries. One subject of considerable interest is the role of diet in heart disease. Due to the fact that diets are so different around the world, it was deemed of particular interest to understand which particular diets were associated with disease. However, the latest WHO health report uncovered a surprising focus, the foods which are associated with the reduction of disease. There was one stand-out food which was grapeseed oil. The study demonstrated that on average, those who consumed 100ml or greater of grapeseed oil per month were 23 times less likely to suffer from coronary heart disease before the age of 55 than those who did not. There were some other foods associated with the reduced risk including jalapeño peppers and avocado, but grapeseed oil was by far the strongest association. Therefore, the report concluded that consuming 100ml of grapeseed oil was highly recommended to prevent coronary heart disease.

Which of the following expresses the strongest flaw in the above report?

A. Grapeseed oil is unavailable in large areas of the world.
B. It implies a causal relationship between grapeseed oil consumption and reduced risk of heart disease.
C. It implies that the consuming of other foods to prevent heart disease is not important.
D. It did not focus on avoiding foods which cause heart disease.
E. It did not take into account the burden of disease in those over 55 years of age.

Answer _____

Q32   In the UK, famous and successful individuals are sometimes criticized for activities in their personal life. This was never more obvious than in the case of Sir Richard Branson, owner of the Virgin Group of companies. Since this group owns an international airline, some would think that Sir Richard would be forgiven for his many unsuccessful attempts to circumnavigate the globe in a hot air balloon. However, the majority of people find this behaviour curious, and in some cases as a flagrant act of irresponsibility. Not only is Sir Richard the head of a corporate empire, with employees ranging in the tens of thousands, he is also a father and husband. What on earth would happen if one of his high-risk adventures were to go wrong? Worse still, his actions inspire other successful individuals to seek danger in sky-diving, base-jumping and other activities. Being successful should not lead to irresponsibility, but rather the growth of responsibility and the avoidance of risk where possible.

Which of the following, if true, most significantly weakens the above argument?

A. Sir Richard has made a will for his dependants and provisions for his companies in the event of an accident.

B. Successful individuals are likely to seek a challenge outside of the workplace.

C. Studies have demonstrated that risk-taking behaviour is a key characteristic of successful businessmen.

D. Insurance policies against injury or death in high-risk pursuits can be obtained by individuals.

Answer

Q33 The role of short-sightedness and the need for glasses in contact sports is often overlooked. Contact lenses are a simple solution for this problem in modern times, as is laser surgery. However, before cheap and readily available contact lenses, those suffering from short sightedness were forced to wear glasses. Having a metal or plastic frame holding glass onto one's face is certainly enough to put one off from certain sporting activities. Just consider football where using one's head to strike the ball is an important part of the game. Who would want to risk damaging expensive glasses, or worse still, risking glass-injury to the eye? Historical data backs up this theory. Asia, the region whose population suffers from the highest proportion of short-sightedness, have also been lowly ranked in national football rankings, never breaking into the top 30 teams. However, only a few years after the advent of cheap and reliable silicone hydrogel contact lens in 1998, teams such as Korea rose in their international rankings, coming to prominence by making the World Cup quarter finals in 2002. This shows that advancing technology has the potential to equalize every human in the world when it comes to sport.

Which of the following, if true, would most seriously weaken the above argument?

A. Cheap plastic frames and shatter-proof lenses from 20 years ago present little hindrance in contact sport.

B. The average height of football players from Asia is 5cm shorter than those from the West.

C. Other sports in Asia such as badminton and table tennis are more popular than football.

D. There was considerable refereeing inconsistency and controversy in the 2002 World Cup.

E. Countries where laser surgery is popular do not perform well in their international football ranking.

Answer [   ]

Q34 When it comes to the use of liquid sunblock on holidays, the scalp may not be the most obvious place in need of protection, as it is partially shielded by the natural barrier of hair overlying it. Nevertheless, people tend to put sunblock lotion on the rest of their bodies to give them protection from UV rays, and therefore the incidence of scalp sunburn is very high. Scalp burns made up 40 per cent of sunburn cases in 2010, with the next nearest being nose (22 per cent) and ears (12 per cent). We would all do well to remember to bring a cap!

Which of the following is a conclusion which can be safely drawn from the above passage?

A. The scalp is biologically the most vulnerable area of the body to sunburn.
B. Hair is less effective at preventing burns than liquid sunblock because it does not prevent UV rays passing through.
C. Exposed areas of the body which are not often clothed make up the majority of sunburn cases.
D. People dislike putting sunscreen on their head as it can make the hair greasy.
E. Sunblock use and location is the key factor in sunburn distribution.

Answer ⬚

Q35 In the infamous 'Lightning Alley' in Florida, US, the chance of being struck by lightning is 1 in 12 thousand per metre of road travelled. If one spent 20 minutes in this region, what is the absolute difference in probability of being struck between a person who runs at 8 km per hour, and a person who walks at 2 km per hour?

A. 12 per cent
B. 14 per cent
C. 16 per cent
D. 18 per cent
E. 20 per cent

Answer ⬚

Section 2 Scientific knowledge and applications

Mock test 14

27 questions
Time allowed 30 minutes
No calculators

Q1   Infective endocarditis is a disease which is caused by bacterial infection of the valves of the heart, and can be 'seeded' from sources of infection. If the needles of an intravenous drug user are contaminated with bacteria, which valve is most likely to be the first to be affected?

    A.   Aortic valve
    B.   Tricuspid
    C.   Bicuspid
    D.   Pulmonary

Answer _____

Q2   Calcium hydrogen carbonate $Ca(HCO_3)_2$ is a buffer in the body. How many moles of oxygen are present in 0.5 mole of $Ca(HCO_3)_2$?

    A.   0.5
    B.   2.0
    C.   1.5
    D.   6.0
    E.   3.0

(hint: atoms)

Answer _____

Q3   Two children throw rocks into the air at the same instant. The stronger one launches it at an initial velocity of 30m/s. The weaker child launches it at 14m/s. What is the difference in the time at which the rocks reach a velocity of 10m/s. $(g = 10m/s^2)$

    A.   0.4 seconds
    B.   0.8 seconds
    C.   1.1 seconds
    D.   1.3 seconds
    E.   1.6 seconds

Answer _____

Q4   Regarding the process of decay and decomposition:

i)   Increasing temperature
ii)   Increasing dryness
iii) Increasing available oxygen

Which of the above will always result in the increase of the rate of decomposition?

A. i only
B. ii only
C. iii only
D. i and ii only
E. ii and iii only
F. All of the above

Answer [   ]

Q5   Which of the following is the best expression of the theory of evolution by natural selection?

A. Individuals with the most breeding capability are most likely to pass on their genetic material.
B. Individuals with characteristics most suited to the environment are most likely to breed successfully and pass on their genetic material.
C. Individuals with characteristics of survival are able to pass on those survival characteristics to future generations.
D. Individuals with characteristics suitable for the current time period may not necessarily benefit their offspring if the environment changes over time.

Answer [   ]

Q6 Which of the following are the products of incomplete combustion?

  i)   CO
  ii) CH_3CHO
  iii) SO_3

  A. i only
  B. ii only
  C. iii only
  D. i and ii only
  E. ii and iii only
  F. i, ii and iii

  Answer [＿＿＿＿＿]

Q7 A car of mass 1000kg is travelling at 8m/s. Its driver then accelerates at 5m/s² for 2 seconds. What is the change in kinetic energy?

  A. 115000 J
  B. 130000 J
  C. 155000 J
  D. 180000 J
  E. 210000 J

  Answer [＿＿＿＿＿]

Q8 Which of the following values for the radius of a sphere results in its volume $(4\pi x)/3$?

  A. $x^{-1/3}$
  B. $3x^3$
  C. $2x^2$
  D. $x^{1/3}$
  E. $4/3x$

  Answer [＿＿＿＿＿]

Q9   Which of the following correctly represents a sequence of events in plant gaseous exchange?

i)   Light, Guard cells flaccid, large stomatal pore, high CO_2 exchange.
ii)   Light, Guard cells turgid, large stomatal pore, high CO_2 exchange.
iii)   Darkness, Guard cells turgid, small stomatal pore, low CO_2 exchange.
iv)   Darkness, Guard cells flaccid, small stomatal pore, low CO_2 exchange.

A.   i + iii
B.   i + iv
C.   ii + iii
D.   ii + iv

Answer

Q10   The upper limit of human hearing is 20,000 hz, and for dogs it is 45,000 hz.

Which of the following combinations of noises are both inaudible to humans but audible for dogs?

	Noise 1		Noise 2	
	Velocity (m/s)	Wavelength (m)	Velocity (m/s)	Wavelength (m)
A	340	55.9	340	82.4
B	350	58.6	350	125.7
C	340	57.4	330	133.3
D	330	69.7	350	120.0

Answer

Q11   In the following diagram, if the area of the square is $4x^2$ and point y is at the midpoint of the square what is the value of A minus B in terms of x?

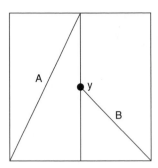

Answer ⬚

Q12   L is a hormone generated by expansion of the gastric wall, which acts by suppressing the desire to intake food. Therefore you might expect mice with the L gene knocked out to be:

A.   Increased mass
B.   Decreased gastric expansion
C.   Decreased mass
D.   Increased gastric expansion

Answer ⬚

Q13   A train of 10×10^4 kg is travelling at 50m/s when the driver sees a vehicle on the rails. Unfortunately, the brakes cannot be engaged, so the driver shuts off the engine immediately before collision. The vehicle on the rails exerts an average stopping force of 50×10^3 N on the train. How far does it travel until it comes to rest?

A.   1.9 km
B.   2.5 km
C.   3.1 km
D.   4.2 km
E.   6.1 km

Answer ⬚

Q14 Which of the following are endothermic reactions?

    i)   Combustion
    ii)   Thermal decomposition of calcium carbonate
    iii)   Neutralisation reactions between acids and alkalis
    iv)   Electrolysis
    v)   Oxidation of iron

    A.   i and iii
    B.   ii and iii
    C.   ii and iv
    D.   iii and iv
    E.   iii, iv and v
    F.   i, ii and v

Answer

Q15 Simplify $(4\times10^{-11})(8.1\times10^{6})$ in scientific notation.

Answer

Q16 A standard fitness test requires users to perform a 'dead lift' by lifting 80kg of weights vertically through 1.3m, then dropping the weight and repeating it as many times as you can in 1 minute. The record number of dead lifts in one minute in a particular gym is 32. Considering only the energy involved in lifting, what is the power of this athlete? ($q = 10$ m/s^2)

    A.   480.6 W
    B.   502.4 W
    C.   520.8 W
    D.   530.5 W
    E.   554.7 W

Answer

Q17 Regarding different cell types in the body:

Type	Function	Characteristic feature
Red blood cell		No nucleus
	Produces antibodies	Has nucleus
	Produces insulin	
		No nucleus
Bacterium cell	Pathogen	

i)   Gland cell
ii)   White blood cell
iii) Reproduction
iv)   Transport oxygen
v)   Platelet
vi)   Cell wall
vii) Sperm cell
viii) Clotting
ix)   Has nucleus

Which of the above does not fit into the above table?

A. vi and ix
B. vii and iii
C. i and v
D. v and viii
E. vi and iii

Answer

Q18 There is a leakage of radioactive material in a school laboratory which occurs at precisely 10am on May 10th 2015. Students make the following measurements of radioactivity in the classroom:

Time and day	Counts per minute
May 10th, 10am	1728×10^3
May 11th, 2am	432×10^3

The safe threshold for entering the classroom is 54×10^3 counts per minute. When will the students be able to re-enter the classroom?

A. May 12th, 8pm
B. May 13th, 2am
C. May 13th, 10am
D. May 13th, 4pm
E. May 13th, 8pm

Answer [   ]

Q19 What is the combined total of protons, neutrons and electrons in Cu^{2+} cations?

$$^{63}_{29}\text{Cu}$$

A. 90
B. 93
C. 95
D. 97

Answer [   ]

Q20 Playing a particular video game involves watching a screen for the emergence of an 'enemy', followed by moving the controller in the player's hands so that it points to the enemy, followed by pressing the trigger.

Which of the following correctly represents the biological sequence of this game?

A.   Retina-motor neurone – synapse – sensory neurone – brain.
B.   Sensory neurone – synapse – brain – motor neuron – effector muscle.
C.   Retina – spinal cord – brain – motor neurone – effector muscle.
D.   Sensory neurone – relay neurone – brain – relay neurone – effector muscle.
E.   Retina – sensory neurone – brain – motor neurone – effector muscle.

Answer ☐

Q21 Simplify $(125x^3/27a^{-3})^{-1/3}$

Answer ☐

Q22 A parachutist of mass 80kg is dropped from a plane at 5,000m altitude. He drops for 10 seconds before opening a parachute. 3 seconds after the parachute opens, his altitude is 4177.5m. What is the negative acceleration exerted on the parachutist by his parachute? $(g = 10m/s^2)$

A. $2.2 m/s^2$
B. $4.3 m/s^2$
C. $5.0 m/s^2$
D. $6.2 m/s^2$
E. $7.1 m/s^2$

Answer ☐

Q23 Which four structures of the cell correspond to the following processes:

i)   Control of cellular activity
ii)   Protein synthesis
iii) ATP generation
iv) The majority of chemical reactions

A.   DNA, ribosomes, chloroplasts, vacuoles
B.   Nucleus, ribosomes, mitochondria, cytoplasm
C.   Nucleus, cytoplasm, mitochondria, ribosomes
D.   Ribosomes, cytoplasm, chloroplasts, nucleus
E.   DNA, ribosomes, mitochondria, nucleus

Answer ☐

Q24   Which of the following are covalently bonded compounds?
   i)   Potassium Chloride
   ii)   Hydrogen Chloride
   iii) Potassium Iodide
   iv)   Calcium Chloride
   v)   Sodium Fluoride

   A.   i only
   B.   ii only
   C.   iii only
   D.   iv only
   E.   v only
   F.   None of the above
   G.   All of the above

   Answer [   ]

Q25   There are 10 boys and 6 girls in a gym class. If one is picked at random, followed by another, what is the probability that there is one girl and one boy in the pair?

   Answer [   ]

Q26   Regarding haploid cells and diploid cells:

   i)   Gamete
   ii)   Embryo
   iii) Sperm
   iv)   Zygote
   v)   Egg
   vi)   Stem cell

   Which of the following are diploid?

   A.   ii and vi
   B.   i and v
   C.   i, ii and iv
   D.   ii, iv and vi
   E.   iv, v and vi

   Answer [   ]

Q27 $NH_4Cl(s) \leftrightarrow NH_4^+(aq) + Cl^-(aq)$ (H = +3.5 kcal/mol)

Which of the following will result in left-shifting of the equation?

A.   Adding NaCL
B.   Increase in temperature
C.   Decrease in temperature
D.   Adding H_4NONH_3

Answer   [   ]

Section 3 Writing task

Mock test 15

Choose one question
Time allowed 30 minutes; you have one side of A4 paper.
No dictionaries

1. Science is the great antidote to the poison of enthusiasm and superstition

Explain what the author means by antidote. Do you think this is always the case? To what extent is the author's position defensible?

2. The best way to reduce the cost of medical care is to reduce the illness (Arlen Spencer)

Explain what the author is suggesting about the state of medical care. Is this always the case? Construct a balanced argument with examples to support your point of view.

3. Love is a serious mental disease (Plato)

What does the author mean by serious mental disease? Does his statement have a reasonable basis in science? To what extent might there be parallels between love and mental disease?

4. Doctors who smoke, drink to excess or are overweight cannot effectively advise patients to alter their lifestyles

Why might the author take this position? To what extent are her viewpoints valid? Explain how her argument might impact healthcare if it is true.

Answers and explanations

ANSWERS TO REVIEW QUESTIONS

Answers to aptitude review questions: Argument

1   *Answer*: C (C offers an alternative explanation to the (false) premise that nuclear reactors are sited away from population centres on safety grounds).

2   *Answer*: A (A significantly weakens the argument on the basis that carbon is taken up (carbon cycle) and the carbon footprint is reduced; D and B are irrelevant because bio-diesel remains an alternative in reducing carbon dioxide emission; C lends support to the argument).

3   *Answers*: A and D (A and D challenge the premises of the argument; B, C and D, even if true, are outside the scope of the argument).

4   *Answers*: B and D (B is the same *method* if beetroot juice is a diuretic and D indicates that the data are valid only for non-hypertensive people; A, C and E may be true but they are irrelevant distracters).

5   *Answer*: B (The key word in the statement is '*but*' because it supports the argument (old bulbs phased out) with the proviso that wind turbines are needed (diversity in modern technologies).)

6   *Answers*: C, A, D, B.

Answers to maths review questions

1   *Answer:* D $(1 - 0.25\pi$; circle $= (\pi \times 2 \times 2)/4 = \pi$; square $= 4$; area of four corners $= 4 - \pi$, so area of one corner $= 1 - 0.25\pi$).

2   *Answer:* E (50 cm²; $AB^2 + AD^2 = 10^2$, ie $2AB^2 = 100$; $AB^2 = 50 =$ area).

3   *Answer:* B ($\sqrt{3}(x^2/4)$; split into two triangles of base length $x/2$, height h, so area $ABC = 2 \times$ (half base $\times$ height) $= 2(0.5 \times (x/2) \times h) = xh/2$, where h is found from the Pythagoras theorem, ie $x^2 = (x/2)^2 + h^2$; so: $h^2 = x^2 - (x/2)^2$, from which it can be shown that $h = \sqrt{(4x^2/4 - x^2/4)} = \sqrt{3}x/2$. Finally, substitute this value of h into the area expression (area $= xh/2$) to give $x\sqrt{3}x/4$).

4   *Answer:* A (Pythagoras theorem: $h^2 = (4 - \sqrt{2})^2 + (2 + \sqrt{2})^2$, ie $h^2 = (16 - 8\sqrt{2} + 2) + (4 + 4\sqrt{2} + 2) = 24 - 4\sqrt{2} = 4(6 - \sqrt{2})$; take the square root to give $h = 2\sqrt{(6 - \sqrt{2})}$).

5   *Answer:* D (36 cm; area $= 3a \times 3a + 1/2 \times 4a \times 3a = 15a^2$; $15a^2 = 60$ so $a^2 = 4$ giving a $= 2$; perimeter $= 6 + 6 + 14 + CD$; $CD =$ hypotenuse h where $h^2 = 6^2 + 8^2 = 100$ so $h = 10$; $10 + 26$).

6   *Answer:* A (2π cm; $<ACB = 2 \times <ADB = 72°$ (using a circle theorem); $72°/360° = 1/5$; $1/5 \times \pi D = 1/5 \times \pi \times 10 = 2\pi$).

7   *Answer:* C (1.1296×10^4; $[6^{2/3}]^6 + [10^{4/5}]^5 = [6^{12/3}] + [10^{20/5}] = 6^4 + 10^4 = 36 \times 36 + 10\,000 = 1296 + 10\,000 = 11\,296$).

8   *Answer:* 1 (divide top and bottom by 3 and express in terms of 8^5:

$$\frac{3 \times (2^3)^5 - 2 \times 8^5}{1 \times 8^5} = \frac{3 \times (8)^5 - 2 \times 8^5}{1 \times 8^5} = 3 - 2 \div 1).$$

9   *Answer:* $x = 4/5$ (($5x - 2)^2 = 4$ so $(5x - 2) = \sqrt{4} = 2$; $5x = 4$).

10 *Answer:* D ($x = 3/2$; $(2x)^8 = (2x + 3)^4$ so $(2x)^2 = (2x + 3)^1$ then $4x^2 = 2x + 3$ and $4x^2 - 2x - 3 = 0$; $(2x + 1)(2x - 3) = 0$ so $2x = 3$ or $2x = -1$; $x = 3/2$ or $-1/2$).

11 *Answer:* 6 20p coins (let $x = 50$p coins and $y = 20$p coins, then: i) $x + y = 15$, $x = 15 - y$; ii) $50x + 20y = 570$, ie $5x + 2y = 57$ so $5(15 - y) + 2y = 57$; $75 - 5y + 2y = 57$; $3y = 18$; $y = 6$).

12 *Answer:* B ($5\frac{5}{7}$; i) $A^3 = 8B^3$ so $A = 2B$; $B = A/2$; ii) $C^3 = 1/8B^3$ so $C = B/2$; iii) box $D = 1\,000$ cm³; side length $= 10$ so $A + B + C = 10$; then $A + A/2 + (A/2)/2 = 10$; ie $4/4A + 2/4A + 1/4A = 7/4A = 10$ and $A = 40/7 = 5\frac{5}{7}$).

13 *Answer:* D ($x^2 - 16 = 0$; $(x + a)(x + b) = 0$; given that $a + b = 0$, then $a = -b$ and $ab = -16$ then $-a^2 = -16$ so $a = 4$ and $b = -4$ to give $(x + 4)(x - 4) = 0$ and finally $x^2 - 16 = 0$).

14 *Answer:* C (1st: $\frac{13}{52}$; 2nd: $\frac{12}{51}$; $\frac{13}{52} \times \frac{12}{51} = \frac{13}{13} \times \frac{3}{51} = \frac{1}{17}$).

15 *Answer*: D ($- 4 \leq x \leq 1$; $x(2x + 6) \leq 8$; i) ÷ 2: gives $x(x + 3) \leq 4$; then ii) expand: $x^2 + 3x \leq 4$; iii) re-arrange: $x^2 + 3x - 4 \leq 0$; factorize: iv) $(x\ 1)(x\ 4)$, adding signs to give $(x - 1)(x + 4)$; finally sketch $y = x^2 + 3x - 4$, using the roots from the factored expression, ie when $y = 0$, $x = +1$ or -4 and when $x = 0$, $y = -4$.

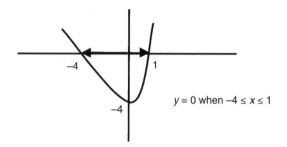

$y = 0$ when $-4 \leq x \leq 1$

16 *Answer*: A $((ac - b)/(a - 1)$; i) cross-multiply: $(y - c) = y - b$; ii) expand: $ay - ac = y - b$; iii) collect y terms: $ay - y = ac - b$; iv) factorize and re-arrange to leave y on its own: $y(a - 1) = ac - b$ so $y = (ac - b)/(a - 1))$.

17 *Answer*: E (sin 270 = cos 180; these are both equal to $- 1$; the trough of the cosine wave is 90° behind the trough of the sine wave; the cosine wave peaks at +1 on the *y*-axis).

Answers to physics review questions

1 *Answer*: 1.25 m ($s = ut + 1/2\ at^2$; $a = g = 10$; $u = 0$; $h(s) = 5t^2 = 5 \times 0.25 = 1.25$).

2 *Answer*: 50 metres (2.5 seconds in flight; 2.5 s $\times$ 20 m s^{-1}).

3 *Answers*: A = gravitational force = 100 N; B = normal force = 100 N; C = friction force = $100 \times 0.2 = 20$ N; D = applied force = 20 N. (The applied force can only be derived from the fact that the object is in constant velocity, and therefore must equal the frictional force.)

4 *Answer*: D: 10 m s^{-2} (B and C are speeds, not accelerations, so this leaves only A and D as possible answers. The acceleration due to gravity (g), which is 10 m s^{-2}, applies to all objects falling to earth, irrespective of their mass (and the speed at which they are thrown). The acceleration of the ball relative to the parachutist is also 10 m s^{-2} because he is not accelerating (terminal velocity reached; weightlessness), ie D).

5 *Answer*: 2.4 kW ((6000 kg $\times$ 10 N $\times$ 2 m) ÷ (50 s $\times$ 1000)).

6 *Answer*: 100 m s^{-1} ($PE_{lost} = KE_{gained}$, ie $mgh = 1/2\ mv^2$ which gives $v^2 = 2gh = 2 \times 10 \times 500 = 10\ 000$ so $v = \sqrt{10\ 000} = 100$).

7 *Answer*: 48 km (work done by scooter = $F \times d = 100$ kg $\times$ 10 N $\times$ 10 per cent $\times$ $d = 100d$ joules; work done by batteries: volts = joules per coulomb, ie joules = volts × coulombs = $24 \times 2 \times 10^5$; hence $100d = 48 \times 10^5$ metres so $d = 48 \times 10^3$ m = 48).

8   *Answer*: B (130 cm from $v = f\lambda$; or work with the units 260 Hz = 260 s^{-1} and v = 338 m s^{-1} so length (m) = 338 m s^{-1} ÷ 260 s^{-1} = 1.3 m).

9   *Answer*: 2 m s^{-1} (action and reaction are equal (Newton's third law) momentum of the bullet = momentum imparted to the gun (choose convenient units, both sides the same); $0.03 \times 400 = 6 \times V$; $V = 3 \times 4 \div 6 = 2$ m s^{-1}).

10   *Answer*: B (2.3 kW; $V = IR$ so 230 = $I.23$ giving I = 10 ohm; power = I^2R).

11   *Answer*: 540 kilojoules (3 kW = 3kJ s^{-1}; 3 kJ s^{-1} × (3 × 60 s) = 9 × 60 kJ).

12   *Answer*: D (J and L; H = uniform (constant) velocity; I = uniform (constant) acceleration; J = increasing velocity = *acceleration*; K = stationary; L = increasing velocity = *acceleration*; M = uniform (constant) velocity; H and M could also be a pair, as could I and L or I and J, but these are not answer choices).

Answers to chemistry review questions

1   *Answer*: B (atomic number = 14 protons = 14 electrons; atomic mass = protons + neutrons = 30; 30 − 14 = 16 neutrons; only the number of neutrons changes in isotopes).

2   *Answer*: C ($C_3H_6O_3$; divide by mass numbers 12, 1 and 16 to give 3:6:3).

3   *Answer*: C (2.4; 200 ml of 1.0 M HCl = 0.2 moles HCl, which consumes 0.1 moles of carbonate (leaving 0.4 moles unreacted), ie the acid is the limiting reactant).

4   *Answer*: a = 6, b = 6, c = 6 (ie all 6; carbons first: 6 CO_2 (b = 6); then hydrogens: 6 H_2O (c = 6); finally oxygen ('on its own'), we need 12 + 6 − 6 to balance the sides, ie 6 CO_2 (a = 6).

5   *Answer*: B (the oxidation states of H and F in forming the compounds are: H = +1, F = −1, and the sum of the oxidation states (oxidation numbers) equals zero for a neutral compound: CF_4 (+4), CH_4 (−4), C_2H_6 (−3), CF_3 (+3), C (0); the lowest of these is −4 in CH_4 (C is −4 and H is +1).

6   *Answer*: D (molecular mass NaCl = 23 + 35.5; so 9 g = 9 ÷ (23 + 35.5) moles NaCl; 1 mole NaCl contains 1 mole of Na).

7   *Answer*: C (there are four positive sodium ions on both sides of the equation which balance the negative charges, so the silver thiosulphate complex on the right-hand side carries no charge (Ag^0); so Ag^{+1} (as AgBr) is reduced to Ag^0, elemental silver, complexed).

8   *Answer*: E (lower the temperature to move the equilibrium to the right in an exothermic reaction and increase pressure because 3 moles become 2 moles. A catalyst increases the rate).

9   *Answer*: E (0.0001 M KOH: pOH = $-\log_{10}$ 0.0001 = 4 so pH = 14 − 4 = 10).

10   *Answer*: A, B, D, C (i = oxidation (A); ii = reduction (B); iii = O_2 (D);
      iv = Cu deposits (C)).
11   *Answer*: T, F, F, T, T (A = true; (3 phases (solid, liquid and gas) and 2 phase
      changes (solid to liquid; liquid to gas); B = false (temperature is below 273
      K/0 °C; the freezing/melting point is at ii); C = false (boiling point is at iii);
      D = true (373 K = 100 °C); E = true (100 K rise from 0 °C to 100 °C)).
12   *Answer*: C, B, G, I, E (i = $C_{10}H_{22}$ (C); ii = C_8H_{18} (B); iii = C_2H_4 (G);
      iv = Br_2 (I); v = $C_2H_4Br_2$ (E)).

Answers to biology review questions

1   *Answer*: D (3:1; Punnett square: two Tt plants: TT, Tt, Tt = 3 tall; tt = 1 short).
2   *Answer*: B (Bb, bb; autosomal recessive; hence has to be bb to be affected).
3   *Answer*: A (AA, Aa, aa; autosomal dominant; hence AA or Aa = affected
     parent (male), aa = unaffected parent (female), Aa = affected child (daughter)
     and aa = unaffected child (son)).
4   *Answer*: E, G, J, K, F, D, H (i = autonomic (E); ii = rods and cones (G); iii = optic
     nerve (J); iv = efferent (K); v = ciliary (F); vi = distant (D); vii = convex (H)).
5   *Answer*: C (a surge in LH triggers ovulation, then progesterone rises to
     maintain the pregnancy).
6   *Answer*: D (most nutrients are absorbed in the small intestine; the pancreas
     releases enzymes to speed up the breakdown of food and an alkaline fluid to
     neutralize stomach acid).
7   *Answer*: B (3 genotypes: AA, Aa and aa, and 2 phenotypes (inherited traits),
     ie either homozygous/heterozygous dominant or homozygous recessive).
8   *Answer*: E (the pulmonary artery carries de-oxygenated blood to the lungs;
     ie less oxygen and more carbon dioxide than blood in the pulmonary vein).
9   *Answer*: C (large protein molecules and red blood cells are not filtered through
     the glomerular capillaries; NB: glucose is reabsorbed in the proximal tubule).

ANSWERS TO MOCK TESTS

Answers to Mock Test 1: Aptitude and skills

1. D	13. B	25. heart murmur
2. E	14. D	26. E
3. C	15. 8,13	27. C
4. 5/8	16. B	28. A and E
5. D	17. 43%	29. B
6. C	18. C	30. C
7. A	19. B	31. B
8. B	20. A	32. D
9. 2	21. D	33. 67
10. E	22. A	34. C
11. D	23. A and D	35. A
12. B, D, A, C	24. E	

1 *Answer*: D (D expresses the main thrust of the argument; A and B are not stated; C is true but misses the main point; E is false).

2 *Answer*: E (E neither supports nor challenges the argument because the people it describes are also failing to maintain their health, but it does not say that they should be discriminated against).

3 *Answer*: C (only C challenges the main conclusion of the argument that nuclear power is both cheap and clean; A, B, D and E are concerned with individual premises).

4 *Answer*: 5/8 (square say $1 \times 1 = 1$; ABC $= 1/2 \times 1/2 \times 1/2 = 1/8$; CDE $= 1/2 \times 1 \times 1/2 = 1/4$; shaded $= 1 - 1/8 - 1/4 = 1 - 3/8$).

5 *Answer*: D (per 100 K $= \times 10$ per million so UK boys + girls $= (3200 + 2000) \times 12 = 5200 \times 12 = 62\,400$).

6 *Answer*: C (UK boys $= 3200 \times 12 = 38\,400$; Spain boys $= 800 \times 10 = 8000$; difference $= 38\,400 - 8000 = 30\,400$).

7 *Answer*: A ($320{:}200 = 32{:}20 = 8{:}5$).

8 *Answer*: B (Spain has the highest boy:girl asthma admission ratio at 2:1).

9 *Answer*: 2 (the thick diagonal remains in a fixed position and the thin line moves a small amount to the right and downward).

10 *Answer*: E (not producing any power (the reason for the claim) makes a power source poor (the claim)).

11 *Answer*: D (D is the best answer because most of the tests are contaminated and therefore of no help in identifying antibiotic sensitivity; in A, waiting for the

results is contraindicated if there is a high proportion of false positives;
B is not to be inferred because the restriction to one antibiotic is not stated;
C should read a low proportion of true positives; E is false).

12 *Answers*: B, D, A, C.

13 *Answer*: B (B correctly identifies the assumption that finding a host is all that is required for pathogenic bacteria to cause an infection; A is false/not stated; C is true but fails to validate the argument; D is a distractor that re-states the argument using 'high probability' in place of the certainly implied statement; E is stated).

14 *Answer*: D (the argument can only leap to its final conclusion by assuming that the medical profession supports the use of cannabis in MS, which is not the same as acknowledging that it can relieve symptoms. A, B and C are all stated in the premises and E is neither stated nor assumed).

15 *Answer*: 8, 13 (0, 1, 1, 2, 3, 5, 8, 13, 21, 34, 55 etc; the Fibonacci series, ie each new term is the sum of the two terms before it).

16 *Answer*: B (76; example method: visualize in three layers each 5 cm deep; top layer $= 0$ without icing; middle layer $= 4 \times 4 = 16$ without icing (and 20 around the outside with icing); bottom layer $=$ same as middle layer $= 16$. Total portions $= 36 \times 3 = 108$; 108 less $16 + 16 = 76$).

17 *Answer*: 43% ($100 - 50 = 50$; $50 \times 1.4 = 70$; $70 \times \% = 100$ so $\% = 100 \div 70 = 10/7 = 142.9 = 142.9\%$, ie $+ 43\%$).

18 *Answer*: C (Speed–time graph: calculate all four *areas* (ie distances apart): $HI = 0.5 \times 20 \times 40 = 400$; $IJ = 0.5 \times 20 \times 30 = 300$; $JK = (0.5 \times 10 \times 30) + (10 \times 30) = 450$; $KL = 0.5 \times 20 \times 30 = 300$).

19 *Answer*: B (15; draw a hexagon and join all the vertices).

20 *Answer*: A (i. School $X = 800 \times 0.25 = 200$ A-grades and school $Y = 660 \times 0.3 = 198$ A-grades, ie *true*; ii. $C + B + A = 66\% \times 800 = 528$, ie *true*; iii. Y pass rate minus X pass rate $= 72\% - 66\% = 6\%$, ie false; i and ii only).

21 *Answer*: D (D is the best answer because it is contrary to the view that chocolate is preferred to healthier food on a cost per calorie basis; A misses the key point altogether; B is counter to the argument; C may be true but it is irrelevant).

22 *Answer*: A (A reflects autonomy, informed choices and the need for 'treatment based on what each individual believes'; B is refuted because the doctor can indicate the preferred option; C and D might be inferred but they do not reflect the passage as a whole).

23 *Answers*: A and D (if A and D are true then the argument is flawed because pensioners can draw on additional sources of income; B does not challenge the 15% of GPD statement and C works out to be no more than 12 per cent of GDP ($4\% + 8\%$ max).

24 *Answer*: E (500 per cent increase $= \times 5$ (5-fold); angina $= 9.1 \div 1.3$ (700%); MI $= 1.7 \div 0.3 = 17 \div 3$ (500+ %); stroke $= 1.8 \div 0.1 = 18 \times 10$ (1800%)).

25 *Answer*: heart murmur (variation = max. minus min. = 2.2 − 1.0 = 1.2).

26 *Answer*: E (none; eg draw three circles that satisfy the description yet challenge the statements).

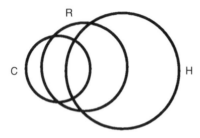

27 *Answer*: C (a true conclusion can be arrived at (accidentally) from false premises; eg replace *aptitude* (the word that links i) with ii)) with *entrance*).

28 *Answers*: A and E (answer A is clearly expressed in the last sentence; answer E must be true when comparing winter and summer deaths if the difference between winter and summer deaths is as stated in the second sentence. B cannot be inferred from the text; C is not the paradox, which is that mortality rates are higher in winter than in summer but not in colder countries compared with warmer countries; D is false because the increasing prosperity refers to warmer countries only).

29 *Answer*: B (B lends the greatest support to the argument because it links mental arithmetic ability with fewer errors; A attempts to undermine the argument; C offers limited support (with no link between over-confidence and errors); D re-states the meaning 'order of magnitude').

30 *Answer*: C (15; 550 − 400 = 150/10 years = 15/yr).

31 *Answer*: B (20 million; reading from the graph: 500 per million in 1995; we have 10 000 giving 10 000 ÷ 500 = 100 ÷ 5 = 20).

32 *Answer*: D (Zak is older than Carl and Leanne is older than Carl so Carl cannot be the second oldest; example of continuum for young to old: Richard, Carl, Leanne, Sarah/Zak).

33 *Answer*: 67 (T1 = 60 × 0.5 + 72 × 0.5 = 30 + 36 = 66; T2 = 90 × 0.4 + 55 × 0.6 = 36 + 33 = 69; T1 = 2/3, and T2 = 1/3; 66 × 2/3 + 69 × 1/3 = 44 + 23 = 67).

34 *Answer*: C (not A because McDonald's does not have the sole right to the prefix Mc; not B because a sign saying Norman McDonald is permissible; not D because it needs to be a food business; C correctly surmises that any attempt to benefit trade by association with the McDonald's chain is defamatory).

35 *Answer*: A (according to the passage any food business placing Mc in front of the name runs a high risk of being forced to change its name; three examples are given in the passage and answer A is consistent with them; answer C is incorrect because the passage indicates a name change with no mention of a fine).

Answers to Mock Test 2: Scientific knowledge and applications

1 *Answer*: C (all three enzymes are produced by the pancreas, and will therefore be produced. Insulin is a hormone which must be in the bloodstream to function, and would be broken down by proteases in the stomach. Amylase is needed as the question states the majority of enzymes are secreted by the pancreas, so even if it is also produced elsewhere, it is still needed).

2 *Answer*: 45 m (two methods: i) conservation of energy (best method): KE lost = PE gained: $1/2\,mv^2 = mgh$, ie $v^2/2 = gh$; $30 \times 30 \div 2 = gh$; $450 = 10h$ so $h = 45$ m.
ii) equations of motion (alternative method): $v^2 = u^2 + 2gh$ with $v = 0$ at the highest point and $g = -10$ m s^{-2} ('deceleration'); $0 = 30 \times 30 + (2 \times -10 \times h)$; $20\,h = 900$ so $h = 45$ m.)

3 *Answer*: D (Right atrium, tricuspid valve, right ventricle, pulmonary artery (via pulmonary valve); 'tricuspid before bicuspid').

4 *Answer*: 9 moles ($2C_8H_{18} + 25O_2 = 16CO_2 + 18H_2O$; $18 \div 2 = 9$).

5 *Answer*: E (27 N; $4 \times 10 = 40$; $40 \times 4 = F \times 6$; $F = 2/3 \times 40 = 80/3 = 26.7$ N).

6 *Answer*: B (48 mph; C, 50 mph is wrong because the time intervals for the two journeys differ. Instead calculate the total time for the round trip and divide this into the total distance for the round trip, ie $240 \div (2 + 3) = 48$).

7 *Answer*: C (carbon forms covalent bonds).

8 *Answer*: D (3 pence; $13 \times 230 \div 1000 \times 4/60 \times 15 = 13 \times 0.23 = 2.3 + 0.69 = 3$).

9 *Answer*: C (chest muscles contract, chest expands, pressure falls, air inspired).

10 *Answer*: J, F, A, C, K, E (i = compound (J); ii = atoms (F); iii = element (A); iv = molecules (C); v = oxidized (K); vi = proton (E)).

11 *Answer*: B (lowest velocity = highest pressure).

12 *Answer*: 15 ($2.5 = (y + 1)^{0.25} + 0.5$; $2 = (y + 1)^{0.25}$ so $2^4 = (y + 1)$; $y = 16 - 1$).

13 *Answer*: C (the concentration of salt is highest at the bottom of the loop of Henle; the diagram indicates that only water leaves at 2, thus concentrating the salt, and that by 4 this concentration has reduced because only salt leaves).

14 *Answers*: C and D (carbon dioxide and hydrofluoric acid form acidic solutions).

15 *Answer*: 10 ohms ($2 + 3 + 5$).

16 *Answer*: E (0%; autosomal recessive inheritance pattern with neither parents of M having an affected dominant allele, ie heterozygous (Aa; Aa) and carriers of a recessive condition such that M must be homozygous recessive (aa) to be affected. His children cannot be affected unless his wife is affected or a carrier).

17 *Answer*: D (carbon monoxide and hydrocarbons are burnt in oxygen; oxygen is removed from nitrogen oxides).

18 *Answer*: D ($F = ma$ for all three couplings; we have $F_i = (20 + 15 + 10) \times 0.4$; $F_{ii} = (15 + 10) \times 0.4$; $F_{iii} = (10) \times 0.4$; ie 18, 10 and 4).

19 *Answer*: 8 £5 notes (let $a = £5$, $b = £10$ and $c = £20$, then $5a + 10b + 20c = 400$ (given) so i) $a + 2b + 4c = 80$; ii) $b = 2a$; $c = b - 6$ (given); substituting ii) in i) gives $a + 2(2a) + 4(2a - 6) = 80$ so $a + 4a + 8a - 24 = 80$ gives $13a = 104$; $a = 8$).

20 *Answers*: C and E (propene is an unsaturated hydrocarbon (C–C double bonds); it reacts with bromine and burns in air to produce carbon dioxide and water)).

21 *Answers*: C and D (eg at $Hb_{50\ per\ cent}$ the partial pressure of oxygen *increases* from approx 27 to 33; at $P_{50\ per\ cent}$ the saturation level drops approx 8% from 83 to 75).

22 *Answer*: D ($x - 3x - 10 \leq 0$; $(x + 2)(x - 5) = y$; $y = 0$ when $x = -2$ or 5 and when $x = 0$ $y = -10$; solution from graph: $-2 \leq x \leq 5$, ie the only possible values of x are $-2, -1, 0, 1, 2, 3, 4, 5$).

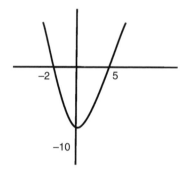

23 *Answer*: C, B, E, F (i = oxidation reaction, loss of electrons (C); ii = reduction reaction (B); iii = Cl_2 (E); iv = H_2 (F). Note that O_2 will form at the anode in a very dilute NaCl solution).

24 *Answer*: D (4, ie two double strands of DNA).

25 *Answer*: A (1.8×10^{18} hertz (Hz); $E = Fh$ so $1.2 \times 10^{-15} = F \times 6.63 \times 10^{-34}$. then $F = 1.2 \div 6.63 \times 10^{19} = 12 \div 6.63 \times 10^{18}$. No further working out is required; only A and E have the correct order of magnitude (10^{18}) and $12 \div 6.63$ must be less than 2 so the only possible answer is 1.8×10^{18} = A).

26 *Answer*: $3\frac{3}{4}$ (($25 + 1/8$) ÷ ($7 - 3/10$) = $201/8 \div 67/10 = 201/8 \times 10/67 = 3/8 \times 10 = 30/8 = 3\frac{3}{4}$).

27 *Answer*: 880 kJ ($4.2 \times 1000 \times (100 - 0) = 420$ kJ to reach boiling point and a further $2.3 \times 200 = 460$ kJ to boil 200 g).

Answers to Mock Test 4: Aptitude and skills

1. A	13. B	25. E
2. B	14. A	26. C
3. C	15. B	27. B
4. D	16. C	28. D
5. 28%	17. D	29. D
6. E	18. D and E	30. E
7. C	19. E	31. B
8. B	20. C, B, D, A	32. C
9. F	21. A	33. B
10. D	22. A	34. A and B
11. E	23. C	35. B and E
12. B	24. D	

1   *Answer*: A (A is a hypothesis that makes sense and is probably true; B is too sweeping a hypothesis; C and D are hypotheses without any foundations and are probably untrue).

2   *Answer*: B (B takes for granted that locally produced food has a lower carbon footprint; A is stated and C, D and E are different arguments).

3   *Answer*: C (more vehicles is a valid alternative explanation for more congestion; A (true or not) is irrelevant as the argument makes no such correlation; B supports the argument; D has no link between economic activity and congestion).

4   *Answer*: D (speed–time graph: the greatest *acceleration*, negative or positive, is given by the steepest *slope*, ie J, and the least *displacement* is the least *area* under the interval, ie M; at I the speed is at its highest and constant so the acceleration is zero).

5   *Answer*: 28% (100 – 20 = 80; 80 – 8 = 72; 100 – 72 = 28).

6   *Answer*: E (E is correct in stating that there is a significant challenge to the argument if 90 per cent of crimes fail to reach court; only a small reduction in crime is anticipated by handing down longer sentences).

7   *Answer*: C (answer C rejects the conclusion that doctors are over-eager to prescribe antibiotics; A explains why doctors might over-prescribe but not why the conclusion is unsafe; B is irrelevant to the argument, and both D and E can be inferred from the argument, so none of these can be the correct answer).

8   *Answer* B. The core argument is that sugary foods cause weight gain. If other sugary foods cause weight gain, this supports this supposition. Other options do not support the argument.

9   *Answer* F

1) Yes, and 2) yes, 3) is not explicitly stated but since the conclusion is that most of the population should avoid it, the negative aspect is deemed to outweigh the positive by the author of the passage.

10   *Answer*: D (two bars have similar heights and two bars have very different heights so not B; A and C are the same so neither of these; ie D pie chart (shortest bar = smallest segment and longest bar = largest segment)).

11   *Answer*: E (2030; *slow method*: you can calculate the gradient from two convenient points (eg 1970 and 1987.5) to see that the line rises by 10 percentage points every 17.5 years; then from 1970 (a convenient point) the line needs to rise exactly 35 percentage points to reach the one-car line; ie (35 ÷ 10) × 17.5 years = 61.25, +1970 = 2031.25; *quick method* (approx.): in the 30 years between 1970 and 2000 the line has risen half the distance it needs (approx 17 per cent) to reach the one-car line and will take another 30 years to hit it if trends continue).

12   *Answer*: B (2/5, ie (initial − final)/initial = (50 − 30)/50); NOT 20% = 1/5).

13   *Answer*: B (400% increase; (final − initial)/initial × 100% = (1/2 − 1/10) ÷ 1/10 × 100% = 4/10 × 10 × 100% = 400%).

14   *Answer*: A (A is an unwarranted assumption because the argument offers no explanation for what it claims other than to state that it is common sense; B is true and cannot be an assumption; C is an implicit assumption of the argument if it is to hold true; D overstates anything that is presumed; E can be discounted on the basis that it refers to the occupants rather than just the driver).

15   *Answer*: B (B is the best answer because it makes no additional assumptions and appears to be the most probable; A and D might be true but there is no evidence given to substantiate these claims; C goes too far in what it claims).

16   *Answer*: C (correlation mistaken for causation (no proven link); only C offers an alternative explanation, ie diagnosis is linked with child's age).

17   *Answer*: D (A is entirely erroneous; B is true as far as it goes; C could be true but is unsubstantiated; E is false because low incomes are a basis for defining poverty; D is the best answer because it acknowledges that few people are living in absolute poverty, with relative poverty and social exclusion described in terms of unequal resources).

18   *Answers*: D and E (D offers an alternative explanation and E contradicts the argument; B neither contradicts nor offers an alternative; both A and C support the argument).

19   *Answer*: E (3.9 and below = 1/4, so 4.0 and above = 3/4; 6.9 and below = 3/4, so 7.0 and above 1/4; 3/4 × 1/4 = 3/16).

20   *Answers*: C, B, D, A.

21   *Answer*: A (Z has lowest proportion without SEN; you need to compare the without/with ratios to find the proportions. V = 700:250 (2.8); W = 250:100

(2.5); X = 400:150 (2.7); Y = 200:50 (4); Z = 600:300 (2). Note that Y has the highest proportion without SEN but the lowest number).

22 *Answer*: A (65 per cent; 'decipher' the question and break it down; the total SEN (Z, Y, X, W, V) = 300 + 50 + 150 + 100 + 250 = 850; the two schools with highest number (not proportion) are Z and V = 300 + 250 = 550; % = 550/850 × 100% = 55/85 × 100 = 11/17 × 100 = 1100/17 = 64.7%).

23 *Answer*: C (4 per cent; step i) SEN with FSM = 850 × 40% = 340; step ii) without SEN with FSM = 426 − 340 = 86; step iii) without SEN = 600 + 200 + 400 + 250 + 700 = 2150; step iv) 86/2150 × 100% = 43/1075 × 100% = 4300/1075 = 4%).

24 *Answer*: D (7; (12 − n) + n + (11 − n) = 18; so 23 − n = 18 giving n = 5, and then Chemistry only 12 − n = 7).

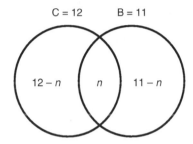

25 *Answer*: E (2.0 L; add x litres of 1.0 molar solution to 0.5 litres of 6.0 molar solution to give (0.5 + x) litres of 2.0 molar solution; total moles of saline are unchanged so write: 1.0x + 0.5 × 6 = 2.0(0.5 + x), giving x + 3 = 1 + 2x; x = 2).

26 *Answer*: C (thiazide diuretic: according to Table 2 the next treatment option would be Step 2, ie add a calcium channel blocker (C) to the ACE inhibitor (A) to give A + C. However, according to Table 1, calcium channel blockers (C) are contraindicated in heart failure. This leaves only the diuretics 'thiazide' and 'furosemide' as answer choices (beta-blockers (B) are not a treatment option in patients with diabetes); finally, thiazide is selected before furosemide according to Table 2).

27 *Answer*: B (calcium channel blocker (CCB): according to Table 2, adding a CCB would be the next treatment option; class B is indicated for angina but not for asthma and is not a treatment option for patients with diabetes).

28 *Answer*: D (29: first round = 32 − 2 = 30 players = 14 matches + 2 unmatched players (automatic win); second round = 8 matches (16 players); third round = 4 matches; fourth round = 2 matches; fifth round final = 1 match. The total number of matches = 14 + 8 + 4 + 2 + 1 = 29).

29 *Answer*: D (£1.05; t + m = 1.10; t − m = 1.00; so 2t + 0 = 2.10, then t = 1.05).

30 *Answer*: E (π/6: sphere: (4π/3)r^3; cube: (2r)^3 = 8r^3; ratio = (4π/3)/8 = π/6).

31 *Answer*: B (B offers an alternative means by which smokers would generate tax revenues if they stopped smoking; A is true but does not link tax and the economy; C is true but introduces new arguments; D is true but is not part of the conclusion).

32   *Answer*: C (C is the only statement that must be false; that patients can make a prior expression of a refusal to have treatment should an emergency situation arise is clearly stated so it cannot be ignored).

33   *Answer*: B (08.50 hrs; Phoebe: $d = st = 3t$; then for Zak: $d = 12(t - 15/60)$; distance d is the same when they meet, so $3t = 12(t - 1/4)$, giving $9t = 3$, ie $t = 1/3$ hr $= 20$ mins; adding this to Phoebe's time gives 08.50 hrs).

34   *Answers*: A and B (A is easily inferred from the fact that disulfiram is indicated to be an *adjunct* therapy; B is more difficult to infer, though the paragraph clearly states that alcohol dependency means that the abuser is unable to stop drinking under any circumstances, making disulfiram therapy entirely inappropriate).

35   *Answers*: B and E (A is incorrect because alcohol abuse is indicated to lead to dependency in some people but not others; C is incorrect because it is alcohol dependency that is the disease process; D is the exact opposite of that stated).

Answers to Mock Test 5: Scientific knowledge and applications

1   *Answer*: F (be careful of your negative feedback loops! FSH stimulates the ovaries to secrete oestrogen. Progesterone (from the corpus luteum) causes negative feedback on both LH and FSH, whereas oestrogen inhibits primarily FSH).

2   *Answer*: B 1.28×10^6 (the table shows that the activity reduces fourfold every day, ie by 2×2 (two-half lives per day); $32 \times 10^4 \times 2 \times 2 = 1.28 \times 10^6 = $ B).

3   *Answer*: C (left atrium, bicuspid (mitral) valve, left ventricle, aorta).

4   *Answer*: E (the oxidation states of H, C and F in forming the compounds are: H $= +1$, C $= +4$, F $= -1$, and the sum of the oxidation states (numbers) equal zero for a neutral compound: H_2O (-2), O_2 (zero), H_2O_2 (-1), CO_2(-2), OF_2 ($+2$); the highest of these is $+2$ in OF_2 (O is $+2$ and F is -1)).

5   *Answer*: 230 N (change in momentum ÷ time taken; $0.046 \times 50 \div 0.01 = 230$).

6   *Answer*: B 2.25π (square $= 3 \times 3$ so circle diameter $= 3$, then area of circle $= \pi D^2/4 = \pi \times 9/4 = 2.25\pi$).

7   *Answer*: C (atomic number $= 36$ protons $= 36$ electrons; atomic mass $=$ protons $+$ neutrons $= 83.8$; $83.8 - 36 = 47.8$ neutrons, and 0.8 neutron is not possible, so there must be isotopes with different numbers of neutrons).

8   *Answer*: C 3 amps (look carefully to see that the battery is across *both* the 2 ohm bulb and the 4 ohm resistor, ie they are wired in parallel. However, you are not asked to calculate the overall resistance so you do not need to use the reciprocal law: 6 volts across a 2 ohm bulb draws 3 amps from $V = IR$; (and 6 volts across a 4 ohm resistor draws 1.5 amps). Check: total current drawn = 4.5 amps and total resistance is given by $1/R_{tot} = 1/2 + 1/4 = 3/4$; $R_{tot} = 4/3$; $V = IR$ so $V = 4.5 \times 4/3 = 1.5 \times 4 = 6$ v (ie checks correct).

9 *Answers*: J, G, C, H, A, E, I, A, D (i = thyroid (J); ii = endocrine (G); iii = metabolism (C); iv = hormones (H); v = pituitary (A); vi = hypothalamus (E); vii = cold (I); viii = pituitary (A); ix = more (D)).

10 *Answers*: B and E (only the alkenes (C_nH_{2n}) are unsaturated and react with bromine by addition).

11 *Answer*: C (Ali: 300 kg m (3000 J) and 15 kg m s^{-1} (150 W)).

12 *Answer*: B 5.67×10^{12} (write all three as 10^{12} ie 5.2×10^{12}, $+ 0.48 \times 10^{12} - 0.01 \times 10^{12} = (5.2 + 0.48 - 0.01) \times 10^{12} = 5.67 \times 10^{12}$).

13 *Answer*: 5500 Pa (or 5.5 kPa; volume = 20 cm × 10 cm × 5 cm = 1000 cm^3; 1000 cm^3 × 11 g cm^{-3} = 11 000 g = 11 kg; 11 kg × 10 N kg^{-1} = 110 N (force). Area = 20 cm × 10 cm = 200 cm^2 = 0.02 m^2. Pressure = force ÷ area = $110 \div 0.02 = 110 \times 50 = 5500$ Pa).

14 *Answer*: A (ultrafiltration (Bowman's capsule), active transport (selective re-absorption), osmosis (water), active transport (salt), osmosis (water)).

15 *Answer*: A (acidosis: excess CO_2 leads to the accumulation of hydrogen ions with a drop in pH).

16 *Answer*: C, B, E, F (i = oxidation reaction (C) with iii (E) chlorine released); ii = reduction reaction (B) with iv (F) hydrogen released).

17 *Answer*: B (method: determine whether abnormality is dominant or recessive (ie not A, autosomal dominant, because neither of the parents can possess an affected dominant gene); B autosomal recessive is possible with both parents carrying the recessive gene (ie heterozygous carriers for the disease); not X-linked because males are not carriers of X-linked conditions).

18 *Answers*: A = gravitational force = 120 N; B = normal force = gravitational force = 120 N; C = applied force = friction force = 30 N; D = net force = 0 (constant velocity = no acceleration).

19 *Answer*: D ($x^2(4 - \pi)/4$; square − circle = $x^2 - \pi x^2)/4 = (4x^2 - \pi x^2)/4$ then factorize to give $x^2(4 - \pi)/4$; NOT answer C, which expands to give $x^2/4 - \pi x^2/4$).

20 *Answers*: B, E, D, B, H (i = boiling points (B); ii = hydrocarbon (E); iii = volatile (D); iv = boiling points (B); v = top (H)).

21 *Answer*: E (receptor, afferent/sensory neurone, central nervous system, efferent/motor neurone, effector/muscle).

22 *Answer*: A ($16\pi^2 r$ newtons; $F = ma = 4 \times v^2/r$ where v = distance ÷ time (ie circumference ÷ time for one revolution) = $2\pi r \div 1 = 2\pi r$ so $v^2/r = (2\pi r^2)/r = 4\pi^2 r$ and F is then given by $4 \times 4\pi r^2 = 16\pi r^2$).

23 *Answer*: B 5/6 (four face cards have been removed to leave 48 cards and eight face cards. The probability of drawing a face card is now 8/48 = 1/6 and the probability of NOT drawing a face card is $1 - 1/6 = 5/6$. NB: the question does not ask what is the probability of drawing the four face cards in sequence).

24   *Answers*: A, C, E, H, B, G (i = gene (A); ii = chromosome (C); iii = allele (E); iv = zygote (H); v = genotype (B); vi = phenotype (G)).

25   *Answer*: A (nitric oxide is a compound, not a mixture).

26   *Answer*: C ($x\sqrt{3}$; drawn a diagonal on the base to give two triangles at right angles, ie a base triangle and a second triangle that includes the diagonal line you want. Pythagoras: base diagonal squared = $x^2 + x^2 = 2x^2$; cube diagonal squared = $2x^2 + x^2 = 3x^2$ so cube diagonal = $x\sqrt{3}$).

27   *Answers*: F, F, T, T, T (A = false; 2 phases (liquid, solid) and one phase change between them (liquid to solid); B = false (could be any temperature below 373 K/100 °C; C = true (boiling point reached); D = true; E = true (pressure lower, boiling point lower)).

Answers to Mock Test 7: Aptitude and skills

1. B	13. C	25. B
2. 56%	14. D	26. D
3. E	15. E	27. C
4. B and D	16. A	28. E
5. D	17. B	29. B
6. E	18. C and D	30. D
7. A	19. E	31. F
8. A	20. C	32. D
9. B	21. D	33. B
10. C	22. B	34. B
11. B	23. E	35. D, A, C, B
12. C	24. 3 litres	

1   *Answer*: B (acceleration–time graph: acceleration × time, ie *area* under the interval = *change in velocity*; H and I look the strongest candidates; I = rectangle = $15 \times 30 = 450$ and H = rectangle + triangle = $(20 \times 10) + (0.5 \times 20 \times 20) = 400$); hence I).

2   *Answer*: 56 per cent ($100 \times 1.8 = 180$; $100 \div 180 = 10/18 = 5/9 = 0.5555 = 55.55$ per cent).

3   *Answer*: E (E is the best answer because it is an alternative to the suggested treatment).

4   *Answers*: B and D (B weakens the ethical position of the argument by offering strong ethical reasons in opposition; D weakens the 'nothing position' assumed of placebo treatments; A fails to challenge the argument and C lends support to it).

5 *Answer*: D: ('cause and effect' not proven; a sedentary lifestyle also leads to a weight increase through increased food intake, ie correlation but no causation).

6 *Answer*: E 1/4 (visualize shapes in turn: small square = 1/4 (2/8); rectangle (half the small square) = 1/8; large triangle = 1/4 (2/8); small triangle (half the large triangle) = 1/8; 1 − 6/8 = 1/4).

7 *Answer*: A (Norton, Ningwood and Niton).

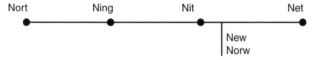

8 *Answer*: A 4.3 per cent (P++ (true+) = 0.005 × 0.9 = 0.0045; P− + (false+) = 0.995 × 0.1 = 0.0995; total positives = 0.0045 + 0.0995 = 0.104 of which 0.0045 are true, ie percentage is given by (0.0045 ÷ 0.104) × 100% = 45 ÷ 1040 × 100% = 9 ÷ 208 × 100% = 900 ÷ 208 = 4.3%).

9 *Answer*: B 28 per cent (estimate bar lengths in (unspecified) units: males 2 + 2 + 2 + 4 = 10; females = 1 + 1 + 4 + 8 = 14; difference = 14 − 10 = 4; 4/14 = 28/98 = 28 per cent (approx) fewer males than female (check: 14 × 72 per cent = 10); note conversely that there were 40 per cent more female deaths than male: 10 × 140 per cent = 14); 'than female' means use female as the starting point).

10 *Answer*: C (add male and female bar lengths by eye and compare ratio of the totals; ie under 65s = 3 divisions (2 male + 1 female); similarly 65–74 total approx 3 divisions (so answers C, D or E), in which case over 85 = 4 male + 8 female = 12 = C only). Put simply, if under 65 = 3, then over 85 = 12).

11 *Answer*: B 8300 (total bar units = 24 (add all bar lengths or tally column C); bar length for females over 85 = 8 units (7.9) = 1/3 of all deaths = approx 8333. Put simply, the female over-85 bar is one-third of the total lengths).

12 *Answer*: C (52 million; 25 000 = 0.048 per cent so 100 per cent = 25 000 ÷ 0.048 × 100 per cent = 25 million ÷ 0.48 giving 2500 million ÷ 48 = 52 million).

13 *Answer*: C (answer C correctly summarizes the key point of grey power, ie more older voters acting in their own interests).

14 *Answer*: D (D is the best answer because it indicates that there could be *alternative* explanations for aggressive behaviour, so reducing screen violence may not be the *best* way to reduce real-life violence).

15 *Answer*: E (not joining a gym (the reason for the claim) makes us less interested in keeping fit; A and D are too firm and too specific; B and C are distracters that are barely hinted at).

16 *Answer*: A (the paragraph indicates that the *concentration* of PSA in obese men is lower whereas the statement indicates that the *total amount* of PSA in obese men is higher, which at first appears contradictory (answer B). However, the concentration could be lower even if the total were higher, so the statement fails to support or challenge the argument, ie A).

17 *Answer*: B (26 bands: $(0.5)^x = 1$:60 million (given); $(1/2)^x = 1/60 \times 10^6$ and $(1/2)^x = 1/2^x$ (because $1^x = 1$) so $1/2^x = 1/60 \times 10^6$; thus $2^x = 60 \times 10^6$; solve, eg $2^5 = 32$ so $2^{10} = 32 \times 32 = 1024$ and $2^{20} = 1024 \times 1024$, ie > 1 million; $2^{25} > 32$ million; $2^{26} > 64$ million).

18 *Answers*: C and D (A is true (end of whisker); B is true $(6.4 - 3.8 = 2.6 =$ inter-quartile range); C is false (lower quartile = 3.8 marks or less); D is false (*median* mark was 5.2); E is true (upper quartile = 6.4 so three-quarters achieved this mark or below, ie 1/4 achieved more than 6.4); the probability of two students achieving more than $6.4 = 1/4 \times 1/4 = 1/16 = 6.25\%$).

19 *Answer*: E (step i): one sector is half the size of the other, which occurs in columns A, C and E but not B and D (ruled out); step ii) C is not possible because no two sectors are the same, so this leaves A and E; step iii) A is 1/8, 1/4, 1/2 (too big), so not A, which leaves E (1/8 (80), 1/4 (160), 280 (7/16), ie fits).

20 *Answer*: C (2006; children's books (CH) accounted for the smallest *proportion* (fraction) in 2006, whereas adult special interest accounted for the smallest proportion in the other years; 2002 CH is a distracter, ie NOT A).

21 *Answer*: D (57%; greatest diff. = highest – lowest; ie 2002 to 2006: 35 to 55; % increase = $(55 - 35)/35 \times 100\% = 20/35 \times 100\% = 4/7 \times 100 = 400/7 = 57\%$).

22 *Answer*: B (£60 000; 2002 to 2004; estimate £65 000 to £125 000; no other answer is close).

23 *Answer*: E (9; draw a table after noting that 1/4 are fiction and 3/4 non-fiction; 24 are paperbacks and 12 are hardbacks).

	P	H	
F	6	3	1/4
N	18	9	3/4
	24	12	

24 *Answer*: 3 litres (1 drop/3 s = 20 dp/min = $20 \times 0.1 = 2$ ml/min = 120 ml/hr = 120 ml/hr $\times$ 25 hr = 0.12 litres $\times$ 25 = $12 \times 0.25 = 3$ litres).

25 *Answer*: B (a rhombus has two lines of symmetry; the remaining shapes all have one line of symmetry).

26 *Answer*: D (7776; $1^0 = 1$; $2^1 = 2$; $3^2 = 9$; $4^3 = 64$; $5^4 = 625$; $6^5 = 7776$ etc).

27 *Answer*: C (there is a weak positive correlation; the points are not sufficiently close to a straight line for it to be a strong correlation; positive because as one test result increases so does the other).

28 *Answer*: E (3 hours 36 minutes; Paul one-sixth per hour; Julie one-ninth per hour, so together = $1/6 + 1/9 = 3/18 + 2/18 = 5/18$ per hour, ie 18/5 hr = 3 3/5 hr).

29   *Answer*: B (2000; code: A = 0, B = 1, C = 2, D = 3, E = 4, F = 5, G = 6 etc;
DACE = 3024).

30   *Answer*: D (D challenges the hypothesis because it states that atmospheric
temperatures have been higher than they are today without anthropogenic
greenhouse gases).

31   *Answer*: F (Be careful when reading the passage here: Digitalis certainly is
a plant-derived medication, and although Digoxin is in the same class of
molecule, it does not mean it has the same origin. Similarly, it has no bearing
on its molecular weight. It has been used as a poison for some time, not sure
about therapeutically!)

32   *Answer*: D
A is not necessarily true – it is less frequently consumed, but for consumers
the risk may be as severe if not more. B is not true – fruits in the family of
grapefruit interact with P450. C is not definitely true. D must be true in the
same way as grapefruit juice. E is unclear.

33   *Answer*: B (for the argument to hold true, most (prevalent) of the elderly
population must attend their GP; if only a small proportion visit their GP
(eg 10%) the argument is false).

34   *Answer*: B (B seriously undermines the argument if there is no evidence of
harm done).

35   *Answer*: D, A, C, B.

Answers to Mock Test 8: Scientific knowledge and applications

1   *Answer*: 11.1% (2(H) ÷ 18(H_2O) = 1 ÷ 9 = 0.111 = 11.1%).

2   *Answer*: D (2 m s^{-2}; m s^{-1} ÷ s = m s^{-2}; 80 m s^{-1} ÷ 40 s = 2 m s^{-2}).

3   *Answer*: A (pharynx, oesophagus, stomach, small intestine, large intestine).

4   *Answer*: E (high electron affinity (strong acceptor of electrons, forming F^-;
the most electronegative element); strongly oxidizing (more than O_2) and
therefore readily reduced (oxidation number decreases 0 to −1);
most non-metallic element).

5   *Answer*: B (0.5 amp; $1/R_{parallel}$ = 1/6 + 1/12 = 3/12; $R_{parallel}$ = 12/3 = 4;
then R_{series} = 4 + 2 = 6, and V = IR so I = V/R = 3/6 = 0.5).

6   *Answer*: C (43/8 ÷ 5/4 = 43/8 × 4/5 = 43/2 × 5 = 43/10 = 4.3).

7   *Answer*: D (2g/5g = 40%; 64/(64 + 32 + 4 × 16) = 64/160 = 4/10).

8   *Answer*: A (13 m s^{-1} east; i) the relative velocity method only works for elastic
collisions: $v_1 - v_2 = u_2 - u_1$ taking care to include the negative sign in front of
velocities to the west (right to left): $u_2 - u_1 = -8 - (6) = -14$ so $v_1 - v_2 = -14$;
and $v_1 = -1$ (given), ie $v_2 = -1 + 14 = +13$ m s^{-1}; ii) conservation of momentum

method applies to all collisions: $m_1u_1 + m_2u_2 = m_1v_1 + m_2v_2$ so $3M \times 6 + M(-8) =$ $3Mv_1 + Mv_2$; $18 (-8) = 3v_1 + v_2$ (cancelling M's) so $3v_1 + v_2 = 10$; $v_1 = -1$ (given), which gives $v_2 = 10 - (-3) = +13$ m s^{-1} as in i); iii) kinetic energy is conserved in perfectly elastic collisions so: $(m_1u_1^2 + m_2u_2^2) = (m_1v_1^2 + m_2v_2^2)$ (cancelling the 1/2 both sides), noting that energy is a scalar ($\pm v$ squared is always positive), so: $3M(36) + M(64) = 3M(1^2) + M(13^2)$, ie $108 + 64 = 3 + 169$; $172 = 172$ (ie elastic).

9 *Answer*: C (expire via: alveoli, bronchioles, bronchi, trachea, larynx, pharynx).

10 *Answer*: 5.0×10^{-5} (($32 + 8$) ÷ (8×10^5) = $40 ÷ (8 \times 10^5) = 5 \times 10^{-5}$).

11 A: true (at node C); B: true (for loop ABCA); C: false (for loop ABCDA; $-I_2R_2$); D: false (not a loop).

12 *Answer*: D (900 ppm; 0.2% w/w = 0.2 g/100 g = 2000 g/million g, ie 2000 ppm; $2000 \times 45\% = 900$ ppm).

13 *Answer*: A (25 per cent; father's parents are homozygous brown (BB) and homozygous blue (bb) so he has a Bb phenotype (heterozygous); mother is stated to be heterozygous (Bb). A Punnett square for Bb father and Bb mother shows that bb (homozygous blue) = 25 per cent chance (1 in 4) with three genotypes (BB, Bb and bb).

	B	**b**
B	BB	Bb
b	Bb	bb

14 *Answers*: B, H, J, C, F (i = base (B); ii = $14 - 2 = 12$ (H); iii = turns litmus blue (J); iv = salt (C); v = 7 (F)).

15 *Answer*: E (v; electric field lines (vectors) radiate outwards from both positive charges; the magnitude is greatest near to the stronger 2C charge and reduces between the charges because like charges repel).

16 *Answer*: C (the father is X^aY; A can be ruled out (dominant A = expressed) as can B (no dominant a = not expressed); D can be ruled out (Y linked); this leaves C and E. Try a Punnett square for X^AY and X^AX^a; unaffected daughter homozygous).

	X^A	X^a
X^a	X^AX^a	X^aX^a
Y	YX^A	YX^a

17   *Answers*: J, I, E, B, G (i = distillation (J); ii = smallest molecules (I);
iii = condensing (E); iv = largest molecules (B); v = least flammable (G)).

18   *Answer*: D (120 V, 15 amps; power in (VI watts) = power out (if 100% efficient)
= 1800 W, so only answers D and E are possible; secondary coil has ×2 more
windings than primary coil so voltage stepped up (×2) not down, ie 240 V).

19   *Answer*: B (–4; $(x - 2)(x + 2) = y$ satisfies $y = 0$ when $x = 2$ or –2; so when
$x = 0$, $y = -2 \times 2 = -4$).

20   *Answer*: C (increased CO_2 shifts the equilibrium to the right and the *buffer*
maintains the pH at 7.4).

21   *Answer*: D (ii must be protein because this is the only substance not to be
filtered out, ie leaves choices B, D and E; iii useful substances are
re-absorbed, ie glucose in C or D, hence D).

22   *Answer*: B (0.5 cm; A = 16B, B = 9C so A = 16 × 9C = 144C, ie area C = area
A/144 and diameter C = diameter A/$\sqrt{144}$ = diameter A/12 = 6/12 = 0.5;
the diameter of a circle is proportional to the square root of its area).

23   *Answer*: A (there are four copies at the start of mitosis (in prophase), ie two
copies from each parent, but there are no copies immediately the cells
separate).

24   *Answers*: D, F, H, B, G (i = oxygen (D); ii = hydrogen (F); iii = half (H),
$H_2O = H_2 + 0.5O_2$); iv = decreases (B); v = increase (G)).

25   *Answer*: C (12 s; Q = CV = 0.1 × 12 = 1.2 coulombs = 1.2 amp for 1 second or
1 amp for 1.2 seconds; we have 100 mA (0.1 amps), hence takes 12
seconds).

26   *Answer*: D ($y^2(x^2 - 2x + 1) = y^2(x - 1)(x - 1)$ and $9x^2 + 6x + 1 = (3x + 1)^2$;
taking the square root of both sides gives $y(x - 1) = 3x + 1$
so $y = (3x + 1)/(x - 1)$).

27   *Answers*: F, T, T, F, T (A = false; only 1 phase change (liquid to solid);
B = true (remains at temperature ii until complete); C = true (fully solidified
then cools); D = false (impurities depress the freezing point, eg antifreeze);
E = true ('opposite directions' but occur at the same temperature)).

Answers to Mock Test 10: Aptitude and skills

1. C	13. C	25. C
2. 270	14. A	26. E
3. C	15. 23	27. E
4. E	16. C	28. B
5. C	17. C	29. C
6. A	18. D	30. D
7. D	19. B	31. B
8. E	20. C	32. D
9. D	21. D	33. C
10. C	22. D	34. C
11. B	23. A	35. E
12. C	24. C	

1   *Answer*: C (A – Communicating easily = increase productivity? Communicating not easily COULD be normal level of production, not necessarily less; B – Incorrect, the information does not allow us to safely conclude this about his eating choice; C – Correct, Alert = less errors, non-alert = more errors; D – Not necessarily, other factors could be involved; E – Not necessarily, other factors could be involved).

2   *Answer*: 270 (The total for each category can be calculated as follows: $210 - 20 - 30 = 160$; $140 - (20 - 40) = 80$; $80 - 30 - 40 = 10$; Total = 250 independent; $520 - 250 = 270$).

3   *Answer*: C (A – Midfielders are fans of Messi and Robben, but not necessarily any others; B – Some like Ronaldo, some like Bale, not necessarily both; C – Correct, Defenders all like Messi and Neymar, and also some like Robben so it must be true; D – There is no specific comment on this; E – Certainly Messi, but since some like Ronaldo and some like Bale, this is not necessarily true).

4   *Answer*: E (Coleen still has 14 minutes, and 7 miles remaining, giving her $V = 0.5$ miles per minute = 30mph. 40miles in 30mph = 1 hour 20 minutes).

5   *Answer*: C (i – This supports the argument; ii – Not specifically related to procedures; iii – Correct, this indicates that significant live patient experience does not protect against complaints, contrary to the passage).

6   *Answer*: A (30 bags × 50 p = £15, £15 × 1.06^3 = £17.87).

7   *Answer*: D (The weakness is that other activities eg sports, crafts, music, might benefit fine-motor skills, when considering video games as 'the best').

8   *Answer*: E (27 + 36 + 18 = 81 = 75 per cent of the total votes. Therefore total number of votes = 81/(¾) = 108; 108 – 81 = 27 = votes for Totonic; 36 – 27 (first minus second [two second places in fact]) = 9 votes difference).

9   *Answer*: D (200 cakes/20 = 10 chef-days, 360 cookies/45 = 8 chef-days; Total of 18 chef-days. 18/3 = 6 chefs).

10 *Answer*: C (if the dose is too low, no one is at risk from illegal users).

11 *Answer*: B (use of pheromones as a relaxant beneficial for mating presupposes that a relaxed state of a partner enhances mating).

12 *Answer*: C (A reduction of $1/8^{th} = X \times 0.875$. This figure reduced by 15% = 0.875 × 0.85 = 0.7875. To return to 100% [Change / original amount]. 21.25/78.75 = 26.98 = 27%).

13 *Answer*: C (A – Not necessarily, the university may have instructed the architect on specific points related to student collaboration; B – This is unrelated to the decision; C – Correct, the decision to employ collaboration-enhancing design is based on the idea that it will improve academic performance; D – This does not impact the passage either way; E – The later part of the passage assumes this but the decision of the university to employ the architect is based firstly on C; his specific actions later are based on E).

14 *Answer*: A (this is in the wording – the minimum number is 10 because each normal day, or gym day, is 50–50 chance, so if every 50–50 chance were to be 0, there would only be 2 Mexican days × 5 tacos = 10).

15 *Answer*: 23 (20 days total. 2 Mexican days × 5 tacos; 8 gym days × 0.5 × 2; 10 normal days × 0.5 × 1; total = 23).

16 *Answer*: C (additional supporting data strengthens the line of argument (although does not necessarily prove it definitively – read the question!)).

17 *Answer*: C (Draw these out if you need to!).

18 *Answer*: D (the Russell group makes up 18 out of 35 sponsors – but no information is given about the amount given by each university. It is not clear that many non-European universities contribute. All we know is that 18 are from the UK, and others from around the world, which could include Europe).

19 *Answer*: B (Whitby: 32/128 = 0.25; Ramsgate: 36/131 = 0.27; Elgin: 20/200 = 0.10; London: 165/641 = 0.257; York: 36/136 = 0.265). Tip – eliminate Elgin by eye. Clearly, it's a low percentage.

20 *Answer*: C (school average = 70%; 34 students buy books and score 70% × 1.2 = 84%; 80 – 34 = 46 students score 70%; New average = 46 × 70% + 34 × 84% = 75.95%).

21 *Answer*: D (small towns: 85 + 32 + 12 = 129 books; 129 × 11 = £1419; Large cities: 165 + 36 = 201 books; 201 × 15 = £3015; Percentage difference = 3015 – 1419/3015 = 0.529).

22 *Answer*: D (can be directly inferred from the statement. A – Supports the argument; B – Unrelated to headmaster's line of reasoning that suffering is beneficial; C – Although there is an unspecified health risk, the headmaster does not argue on the grounds that his policy is risk-free. His reasoning of suffering improves perseverance is supported by this; D – The headmaster argues that suffering can improve mental fortitude and perseverance. The study in D directly contradicts this; E – Supports his position).

23   *Answer*: A (key argument is that suffering will benefit students, this undermines it).

24   *Answer*: C (C correctly identifies the unstated assumption (the link) that it is the competing (not just the taking part) that can be psychologically damaging; B re-states the argument from the opposite perspective; A, D and E can be excluded on the basis that they introduce new arguments).

25   *Answer*: C (both groups do well at A level (innate intelligence) and group B's ability to think through unfamiliar problems (thinking ability) can be developed (improved scores) with practice; not D because a poor performance is not indicated in the paragraph).

26   *Answer*: E

27   *Answer*: E

28   *Answer*: B ($114 \times 0.58 = 66.12$ goals; $66.12 / 9 = 7.34$ goals)

29   *Answer*: C (cost% $= 50/212 = 23.6\%$; Goal% $= 9/132 = 6.8\%$; $23.6 - 6.8 = 16.8\%$).

30   *Answer*: D (supporting argument: alternative therapies persist due to effectiveness. If true, this strongly undermines the argument).

31   *Answer*: B (the next line describes the previous eg the 2nd line is 'one 1' = 11; The next is two ones = 21; The next is one 2, and one 1 = 1211; Solution = Three 1's, two 2's then 11 = 312211).

32   *Answer*: D (core conclusion stated, others are supporting or subsidiary points).

33   *Answer*: C (Since the argument is supported by the concept that conventions provide a safe environment, harassment and violence at such events would undermine this theory).

34   *Answer*: C (Chris contributes 150,000 represented by a score of 80; Steph's score of 20 represents ¼ of this, therefore $150,000/4 = 37,500$; Alternatively, $(150,000 / 80) \times 20$).

35   *Answer*: E (Chris total weighted score $= 1760$; Steph total weighted score $= 840$; Arthur total weighted score $= 600$; Total $= 3200$. $600/3200 = 18.75\%$).

Answers to Mock Test 11: Scientific knowledge and applications

1   *Answer*: D (white blood cells perform three main actions against pathogens; ingestion, antibody production and antitoxin production. The first two avoid these actions, whereas the third can be countered by antitoxins under most circumstances).

2   *Answer*: E (citric acid is polyprotic $C_6H_8O_7$ (Triprotic) as it donates 3 protons per molecule during dissociation; Hydrochloric acid (HCl) and Nitric acid (HNO_3) donate one proton per molecule and are monoprotic).

3   *Answer*: E ($V^2 = U^2 + 2as$; $0 = 10^2 - 4s$; $S = 100/4 = 25m$; $40 - 25 = 15m$).

4   *Answer*: A ($5x + 15 = 5(x + 3)$; $x^2 - 9 = (x + 3)(x - 3)$; cancelling these expressions leaves us with $5(x - 3)$ and as $(y - 4)x - 1 = 4 - y$, this becomes $5(3 - x)$).

5   *Answer*: D (Step 4, the production of transmitter molecules, must be produced prior to the AP arriving. They then release, diffuse across the synapse and trigger the AP in the 2nd neuron).

6   *Answer*: A ($V = f\lambda$; $340/500 = 0.68$ m; $1400/500 = 2.8$ m; $280 - 68 = 212$ cm).

7   *Answer*: 8 and 6 (these are the following averages of the digits in order: 19/3, 21/3, 15/3, 16/3, 13/3, 21/3).

8   *Answer*: G (ii would not result in increased reabsorption. i causes high levels of glucose in the blood, and thus high levels of filtered glucose, which results in higher-than-normal glucose absorption, but less net water reabsorption as the highly concentrated filtrate draws water out with it. iii reduces flow through the kidneys, causing less reabsorption of glucose as less is filtered).

9   *Answer*: D

10 *Answer*: B (i – $NH_4Cl \rightarrow NH_3 + HCl$; ii – $2H_2O \rightarrow 2H_2 + O_2$; iii – $CaCO_3 \rightarrow CaO + CO_2$; iv – $Na_2CO_3 \rightarrow Na_2O + CO_2$. Firstly, demonstrate the results of the decomposition reaction. HCL will react with CaO in a 2:1 ratio – $CaO + 2HCl \rightarrow CaCl_2 + H_2O$. It may react with Na_2O in a 1:1 ratio – **$Na_2O + HCl = HO + Na_2Cl$**, in a 1:1 ratio).

11 *Answer*: 16 (the sequence is 'Prime numbers, minus 1': 2, 3, 5, 7, 11, 13 and 17 should always be visible to you!).

12 *Answer*: C (GPE = MGH = 0.12 x 10 x 2 = 2.4 Joules; GPE = KE = $\frac{1}{2}mv^2$; $2.4 = \frac{1}{2}mv^2$; $2.4 / (1/2 \times 0.12) = v^2$; V = $\sqrt{40}$).

13 *Answer*: E (GM crops can have negative effects on insect populations; this is a corollary of i!).

14 *Answer*: B (V = IR; 500 x 0.5 = 250 Volts; P = IV = 125 watts; 20/125 = 0.16).

15 *Answer*: E (Propyne have triple carbon-carbon bonding. All others are double or less).

16   *Answer*: A (both sensory and motor neurones synapse in the CNS. Effectors can be glands eg sweat glands!)

17   *Answer*: $(X + 4)/(X + 6)$

18   *Answer*: D (step-up transformers have high secondary-to-primary ratio. Energy transferred is in kW hours (kWh)).

19   *Answer*: C (Protease works best at a higher temperature and in acidic (stomach) conditions, and lipase in the higher pH environment of the small intestine with the presence of bile. Almost all enzymes and hormones function better under condition 2 (higher concentration + temperature).

20   *Answer*: C (first, write a balanced equation for the reaction

$$2Al_{(s)} + 3CuSO_{4(aq)} \longrightarrow 3Cu_{(s)} + Al_2(SO_4)_{3(aq)}$$

Calculate the moles of copper = 6 g/64 g mol^{-1}
$$= 0.093 \text{ mol}$$

From the equation, the maximum amount of aluminium metal that could be present = $^2/_3 \times$ the amount of copper made, as the ratio of Al : Cu is 2 : 3. Aluminium involved in the reaction = $^2/_3 \times 0.093$ mol = 0.062 mol Aluminium $\times 27 = 1.674$g; Purity = AL in reaction/mass of sample = (1.674 g/4.0 g) $\times 100 = 41.85\%$).

21   *Answer*: E (i – yes, the more conductive a substance, the faster it changes the temperature of the hand feeling it!; ii – yes; iii – Yes; iv – No, due to the bonding, molecules in solid water is less easily rotated, therefore heating less well).

22   *Answer*: B (Meiosis produces haploid cells, at all times after puberty occurs, not only when reproducing).

23   *Answer*: B (increasing temperature and pressure increases reaction rate, as does a catalyst. Increasing the solute of a reactant decreases its concentration, lowering the reaction rate. Remember that increasing surface area leads to increased reaction rates, so dividing solid reactant pieces increases the rate).

24   *Answer*: C (surface area of the vertical walls = circumference x height = $2\pi r \times H$ $= 2 \times 1/2D \times \pi \times H = \pi DH$; Surface area of bottom surface = $\pi r^2 = \pi (D/2)^2$).

25   *Answer*: D (establish the half-life of substance x; Reading the data, you can see that 86/2 = 43, with a time interval of 30 minutes. Therefore, t1/2 = 30 minutes, and therefore the starting amount is twice the value at 30 minutes = $86 \times 2 = 172$).

26   *Answer*: D (individual efficiency: P = IV; $10 \times 240 = 2400$ W; $140/2400 = 0.058$; Power saving = $8 \times 240 = 1920$W; $320 /1920 = 0.167$; $0.167 – 0.58 = 0.109$).

27   *Answer*: D (Separate horizontal and vertical elements. (horizontal) WD = F $\times$ D, $60 \times 100 + 10 \times 20 + 5 \times 40 + 2 \times 60 = 6520$ J. Vertical = MGH. $(60 \times 10 \times 10) +$ $(10 \times 10 \times 2) + (5 \times 10 \times 4) + (2 \times 10 \times 6) = 6520$. $6520 + 6520 = 13040$ J) [notice that because of the incline ratio, both vertical and horizontal measurements are the same].

Answers to Mock Test 13: Aptitude and skills

1. D	13. A	25. E
2. E	14. D	26. B
3. E	15. B	27. A and B
4. B	16. D	28. S
5. C	17. B	29. C
6. C	18. A	30. C
7. B	19. B	31. B
8. B	20. B	32. C
9. C	21. D	33. A
10. B	22. D	34. C
11. C	23. B	35. C
12. A	24. B	

1 *Answer*: D (the key **conclusion** of the passage is that 'we should not believe in the lie that our society is meritocratic' eg 'our society is not meritocratic'; B – This is the opposite of the conclusion; C – The author concludes a reflective belief 'our society is not meritocratic', not a prospective belief 'we should be meritocratic'; D – If people are unsuccessful through their own fault, that is meritocratic. If they are unsuccessful not through their own fault, it is not meritocratic. This exactly mirrors the conclusion of the author; E – Whilst true, this is not a summary of the conclusion of the author. It is common to include additional sentences at the end of passages to distract from the actual conclusion; look out for this trick!).

2 *Answer*: E (Best = W, W, D as the only possible 7 point combination; OK is either = D, D, D or W, L, L but since Terrible = 0 then they cannot have drawn with OK, so OK must be W, L, L; Terrible = L, L, L; Good has W vs Terrible, since Terrible lost all 3 (G = W ? ?); Since OK has one W, and Terrible has 3 Losses, OK must have beaten Terrible; Since OK must be W L L, Good must beat OK; Therefore, Good is W vs OK, W vs Terrible; Best must have beaten OK and Terrible, and therefore drawn with Good, in order to have 7 points. Therefore Good and Best have W, W, L and 7 points each; Therefore = 7 points).

3 *Answer*: E (A – Whether or not wine is fermented using yeast is not stated. Champagne is bubbly because of the fermentation inside glass bottles, not necessarily yeast; B – Close, but the relative health risks of alcohol excess vs tannins and sulphides is not described, therefore it is unsafe to conclude this; C – This is not specifically stated, also both wine and champagne are stated to be harmful in excess; D – Incorrect; E – Correct, they CAN be harmful to health, if drunk in excess as stated due to alcohol).

4   *Answer*: B (There are two methods of approaching this – top down, or bottom up. Top down; maximum of 5 players – First game starts after 25 × 5; 2 hours 5 mins until game starts at 1605. The players can begin reading the rulebook at this time. Therefore the next set of 5 takes another 2 hours 5 minutes, meaning the next game commences at 1810. From 1810 to the end at 1940, there is 90 minutes. The maximum number of players reading the rulebook in this time is 3 × 25 = 75 minutes, with 15 minutes remaining for the game. 5 + 5 + 3 = 13; Bottom up; this method is far faster. The total party duration is; 5 hours 40 minutes = 340 minutes. The last game must have commenced at 340 – 15 = 325 from 2pm. 325 minutes divided by the time it takes to read the rulebook = 325/25 = 13 players).

5   *Answer*: C (the author argues that such feedback should NOT be given, the only justification for which is the risk that there will be a doctor shortage).

6   *Answer*: C (filtering unsuitable doctors represents a positive reason for exposing students to realities of medical life, and therefore represents a weakness in the argument).

7   *Answer*: B (i – If 1/3rd of the incidents involved fans whose team did not make the group stages, it is possible that up to 2/3rds involved fans whose team DID make it. Therefore, this is unsafe; ii – If 1/3rd of incidents involved European fans whose team did not make the group stages, then at least 1/3rd did, and possibly more including non-European teams who did not make the group stages. Therefore, this is safe; iii – This is not necessarily true, although it is theoretically possible that reducing the number of fans in general would reduce violence, it is also possible that having a higher proportion of remaining fans whose team made it past the group stages (remembering they made up 2/3rd of the violent incidents!) could increase the violence. Therefore, this is possible, but not a safe inference).

8   *Answer*: B (Max: 29.3 minutes, Julie: 20.6 minutes, Agatha 21.4 minutes, Shane: 23 minutes).

9   *Answer*: C (7.35 arrival time, minus travel time of 21.4 minutes = 7 o'clock + 13.6 minutes = 7.13 and 36 seconds [converting fractions of a minute]).

10   *Answer*: B (journey time of 20.6 means leaving at 20.6 + 25 = 45.6 minutes to cover 1.1 km = CONVERT TO HOURS = 1.1 (45.6/60) = 1.44).

11   *Answer*: C (Agatha travel time = 21.4 +/– 10 mins = 31.4 mins to 11.4 mins. Distance = 3.5km. (3.5/31.4) × 60 = Min speed in km/hour = 6.69. (3.5/11.4) × 60 = Max speed in km/hour 18.42. Difference = 11.73).

12   *Answer*: A (lowest percentage commission, regardless of fee).

13   *Answer*: A (Step 1 Convert to Dyat (250/6 = 41.67 dyat. Step 2 remove percentage commission: 41.67 – (41.67 × 0.022) = 40.75. Step 3: Remove fee 40.75 – 3 = 37.75).

14 *Answer* = D (The existence of a new way to get semiconductor material onto silicon may or may not result in functioning chips, because as stated, they need to be in 'fine pathways'. This method may, for example, bind the material to the silicon in a dispersed pattern. (This technique of referring to important data early on in a passage is a trick that is sometimes used in the exam – beware!).

15 *Answer*: B (18.75% change in blood volume = class II Haemorrhage = heart rate increase by 22%. $60 \times 1.22 = 73.2$).

16 *Answer*: D (the key sentence is 'as a result of these studies…' and students being recommended the splints is the main conclusion).

17 *Answer*: B (the core tenant of the argument involves 'Inflammation and therefore pain').

18 *Answer*: A ($110000 \times 0.8 = 88000$ = total luxuries; $88000 \times 0.4 = 35200$ absolute spending on truffles; $35200/140000 = 0.251 = 25\%$).

19 *Answer*: B (A – It is not clear if biofuels will be implemented in this way, only the potential is discussed; B – stated as a result of economics; C – not stated; D – not stated).

20 *Answer*: B (supports the view that biofuels will cause environmental problems).

21 *Answer*: D (A – As stated, you the patient can seek a second opinion; B – This does not impact abortions after 24 weeks. Also whilst many may object, this is not all; C – This supports the argument – the conclusion likely to be true if this is the case; D – As stated in the passage – there are strict laws governing abortions. The conclusion that you can get an abortion regardless of the doctor agreeing is untrue – all doctors follow the 1967 Act in deciding if your abortion is legal – they can then object to perform it on religious or philosophical grounds. Therefore, if you do not have a legal reason for having an abortion, as listed, you would not be able to have an abortion; E – This supports the argument, as it is easier to have an abortion).

22 *Answer*: D (15.7% – 150 / (480+100+150+220)).

23 *Answer*: B (McColonel – 160; Burger Ronald – 1.09; KFC – 1.41; Wompy – 1.25).

24 *Answer*: B (Normal meal = 320+120+140+200 = 780 calories total; Salad version = 720 total. 720/780 = 9.3%).

25 *Answer*: E (KFC Drink = 100/100 = 1cal/p; KFC Dessert = 220/170 = 1.29cal/p; Wompy Burger = 300/240 = 1.25 cal/p; Wompy Drink = 120/100 = 1.2 cal/p; Wompy Dessert = 210/100 = 2.1 cal/p [Tip: if the denominator is 100 for several, it is easy to see that dessert stands out as much higher!]).

26 *Answer*: B (ii – provides an alternative reason to why young people prefer magic, thereby undermining the argument; i – Short attention spans would mean that a stimulus holds their attention for a short period, making them hard to distract. This would be another, plausible biological argument for why older people are less susceptible to magic than younger people, therefore supporting the argument; iii – Does not support or refute the argument).

27   *Answer*: A and B (A – The argument is valid if we assume the resources needed for treating both diseases is similar – if one is far more expensive than the other, we cannot argue for that to be the focus on the above reasoning alone; B – Infrequent events which kill large amounts may be outweighed by common, individual diseases affecting thousands each year; C – Although this is similar to B, the role of an individual state does not impact the focus of the organization as a whole; D – Non-medical intervention may have some impact in epidemics via eg quarantine, but equally on individual diseases eg food labelling. It impacts both choices; E – Public perception should not impact the decision making priority of life-saving).

28   *Answer*: S (I and X are easily eliminated because they look the same whether turned upside down or reflected in a mirror; B, C and E do not have rotational symmetry and when turned upside down the left becomes the right, which is then reversed back again on reflection when the right becomes the left, so not B, C or E. S has rotational symmetry and appears unchanged on turning upside down and is thus incorrect after reflection).

29   *Answer*: C (A = 1, B = 2, C = 3, D = 4 etc; every column/row adds to up 12).

30   *Answer*: C (the link between exposure to coding from a young age, and excellence in IT skills is assumed).

31   *Answer*: B (association does not mean causation. B represents this flawed reasoning).

32   *Answer*: C (the argument is that being successful should not lead to irresponsibility; this statement demonstrates that the two are in fact linked).

33   *Answer*: A (this directly refutes the argument that breaking expensive glasses or having glass-injuries are the causes of risk averseness in striking the ball with one's head, as claimed in the passage).

34   *Answer*: C. (This statement is borne out directly from the statistics, as 40%+22%+10% of the sunburns are in areas which fit the description).

35   *Answer*: C (calculating the individual probabilities: 20 mins @ 8kmph = 2.6km travelled = 2600m; 20 mins @ 2kmph = 667m travelled; Probability of being struck by lightning = 2600 × (1/12000) = 0.216 = 21.6%; 667 × (1/12000) = 0.00555 = 5.55%; 21.6% – 5.55% = 16% absolute difference in being struck by lightning (reminder – this is not relative difference)).

Answers to Mock Test 14: Scientific knowledge and applications

1 *Answer*: B (tricuspid valve – this is the first valve met by incoming blood as it enters the heart).

2 *Answer*: E 3 moles ($3 \times 2 \times 0.5$ moles, per mole of compound).

3 *Answer*: E ($V = U + at$; $10 = 30 - 10t$, $10t = 20$, $t = 2$ seconds [strong child]; $10 = 14 - 10t$, $T = 0.4$ [weak child]; $2 - 0.4 = 1.6$ seconds).

4 *Answer*: C (careful here: increasing temperature will increase the rate of reaction, until the point where bacteria die – therefore not 'always'. Increasing moisture levels increases rate of reaction, again until a saturation point. However, increasing aerobic conditions will always enhance the rate of decomposition).

5 *Answer*: B (suitability and successful breeding are the cornerstones of natural selection. Answer C is close, but it really only explains genetic inheritance, whereas B focuses on the probabilistic nature of natural selection as well).

6 *Answer*: D (CO = carbon monoxide from incomplete combustion of hydrocarbons. CH_3CHO = aldehyde from incomplete combustion of ethanol. SO_3 = complete combustion of sulphur ($2S + 3O_2 => 2SO_3$).

7 *Answer*: B ($\frac{1}{2} mv^2$, $500 \times 64 = 32000$ J, $18 \times 18 \times 500 = 162000$ J, $162000 - 32000 = 130000$ J).

8 *Answer*: D

9 *Answer*: D (turgid guard cells open stomata).

10 *Answer*: D ($V = f\lambda$, $330 \times 69.7 = 23001$, $350 \times 120.0 = 42000$).

11 *Answer* $= \sqrt{5x^2} - \sqrt{2x^2} = x(\sqrt{5} - \sqrt{2})$

12 *Answer*: A (increased mass – relief of appetite suppression with result in increased appetite and increased mass as a result).

13 *Answer*: B ($F/M = A$; $A = -0.5$; $V^2 = u^2 + 2as$; $0 = 50^2 + 2 \times -0.5 \times s$; $S = 2500$ m).

14 *Answer*: C (combustion is exothermic, as are most neutralization reactions apart from ethanoic acid and sodium carbonate and rusting. Electrolysis is endothermic, and thermal decomposition of calcium carbonate requires the input of heat and is endothermic).

15 *Answer*: 3.24×10^{-4}

16 *Answer*: E ($WD = F \times D$, $800N \times 1.3m \times 32 = 33280$ J, Power = Energy/time, 33280 J/$60 = 554.7$ W).

17 *Answer*: B (sperm cells are involved in reproduction and have a nucleus. They could not fit in this table).

18 *Answer* $=$ B (Firstly calculate half life, determine how many half lives are needed, 16 hour gap $= 1728 / 2 = 864$, $864/2 = 432$. Therefore 8 hour half life. 5 half lives are needed to get to 54×10^3, therefore 5×8 hours $= 40$).

19 *Answer*: A (atomic mass = protons + neutrons = 63; atomic number = the number of protons (defines the element) = 29 for Cu, with 29 electrons for a neutral atom and 27 electrons for a 2 + cation, ie protons + neutrons + electrons = 63 + 27 = 90).

20 *Answer*: E

21 $\dfrac{[5^3x^3a^3]^{-1/3}}{[3^3]}$ (take a cubed root = $(5xa/3)^{-1}$ = 3/5xa).

22 *Answer*: C (after 10 seconds, S = ut + 1/2at². S = 0 + ½ × 10 × 100 = 500m; Also, V = u + at = 0 + 10 × 10 = 100. From 10–13 seconds; 322.5 in 3 seconds, 322.5 = 100 × 3 + ½ × a × 9, 322.5 – 300 = 4.5a. 22.5/4.5 = 5 = a; Therefore the negative acceleration is 5m/s).

23 *Answer*: B (Cytoplasm = largest area, majority of reactions, others functional).

24 *Answer*: B (HCL. You may be tricked because chlorine's greater electronegativity causes a high degree of polarisation of the bond, so it is highly soluble – but nevertheless the bond is covalent).

25 *Answer*: ½ (if a boy picked (10/16), then the chance a girl is picked is (6/15); if a girl is picked (6/16) then the chance a boy is also picked is 10/15; 10/16 × 6/15 simplifies 5/8 × 2/5 = ¼; 6/16 × 10/15 simplifies to 3/8 × 2/3 = ¼). 1/4 + 1/4 = ½.

26 *Answer*: D (gametes, sperm and eggs are haploid, others diploid).

27 *Answer*: C (if H = +3.5 kcal/mol then the reaction is endothermic, so decreasing the temperature will cause a left-shift).